DIM-MAK'S

12 Most Deadly Katas

DIM-MAK'S

12

Most Deadly Katas

Points of No Return

Erle Montaigue

PALADIN PRESS
BOULDER, COLORADO

Also by Erle Montaigue:

Advanced Dim-Mak: The Finer Points of Death-Point Striking
Dim-Mak: Death-Point Striking
Secrets of Dim-Mak: An Instructional Video

Dim-Mak's 12 Most Deadly Katas:
Points of No Return
by Erle Montaigue

Copyright © 1995 by Erle Montaigue

ISBN 0-87364-826-9
Printed in the United States of America

Published by Paladin Press, a division of
Paladin Enterprises, Inc., P.O. Box 1307,
Boulder, Colorado 80306, USA.
(303) 443-7250

Direct inquiries and/or orders to the above address.

Illustrations are based on *Point Location and Point Dynamics Manual*, by
Cameron and Carole Rogers. Used with permission.

CONTENTS

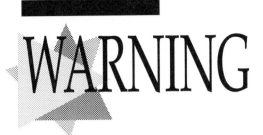

WARNING

The techniques and drills depicted in this book are extremely dangerous. It is not the intent of the author or publisher to encourage readers to attempt any of them without proper professional supervision and training. Attempting to do so can result in severe injury or death. Do not attempt any of these techniques or drills without the supervision of a certified instructor.

The author, publisher, and distributors of this book disclaim any liability from any damage or injuries of any type that a reader or user of information contained within this book may incur from the use of said information. *This book is for academic study only.*

INTRODUCTION

The most amazing things on this earth are the things that we take for granted, the most common things. We go to the movies and look in awe at the computer dinosaurs in *Jurassic Park*, or we watch a martial arts film and say how amazing that kick was. And yet, right under our noses we have the most amazing things ever invented. I go running and just take for granted that my ankles and feet are going to support me, taking such punishment. I look down and see these two miracles of nature working and I stop running. What sort of genius made my ankles? What genius engineer worked out how to put together my feet so that they are able to take such strains? The scientists tell me that evolution caused such wonders to happen by accident! I can't believe that. Who decided, for instance, that bones would be stronger if they were hollow? Never has a solid bone been found, so bones must have been hollow from the beginning. And when we look at the composition of bone, it becomes obvious that bone was not formed by some accident but that some megaintelligent "thing" must have worked it out over many millions of years. Just read the following excerpt from the *World Book Encyclopedia* and tell me if it could have happened by accident.

> BONE: rigid supporting tissue constituting the principal component of almost all adult vertebrate skeletal structures and existing in either dense or spongy form, known respectively as compact and cancellous bone. Bone consists of a chemical mixture of inorganic salts (60 to 70 percent) and various organic substances (30 to 35 percent) and is both hard and elastic. Its hardness is derived from inorganic constituents, principally calcium phosphate and calcium carbonate, with small amounts of fluorides, sulfates, and chlorides; its elasticity is derived from such organic substances as gelatin, collagen, and traces of elastin, cellular material, and fats. . . .

All of that by accident? I don't think so. An intelligence that could work out how to build a human being, or even a blade of grass, is awesome, and such intelligence made we human beings perfect. Everything on this earth was made perfect by whatever it was that made us. But in order for us to stay perfect, we were given certain guidelines within which to stay. We were given the ideal fuel, the ideal way of moving to keep the body healthy, and clean air and water. Well, we've stuffed the latter two of those, but the food and the movement we can do something about. (Actually, we can do something about the air and water, too, if we want to move to where we are able to get such dwindling treasures nowadays.)

The martial arts provide us with a way of moving that is natural and body building. I mean those martial arts that are of the "internal" variety, those that do not force us to move unnaturally, with external tension causing adverse effects upon the chemical makeup of the body.

Taiji, or dim-mak, is one of those martial arts that causes the body to move naturally, only using the right muscles for the job at hand, with every bone, sinew, and muscle moving in coordination. This natural movement allows the body to renew itself more readily (as it should naturally) and get rid of the old in order to grow new tissue. It is in harmony with the Universe, or God, if you like. The whole Universe moves and lives in a certain chaotic way. And this is the same way that the body grows and renews itself. If our mind and body are out of harmony with the Universe, then they will not join the natural chaos and will soon become ill and die. Everything has a life cycle, but we have caused our own to be shortened, simply by being human beings. We live in a totally unnatural environment, which causes us to move, eat, and, more importantly, think unnaturally.

Human beings were not meant to be killers. We were not given the natural weapons to be killers. Animals were given the tools to be natural killers. It is not the way of the human being to hurt or to kill. But look around us and we see that human beings are indeed killing. We not only kill other animals but each other as well. Most of the population of the world has become unnatural—eating unnatural foods, moving the wrong way, and thinking the wrong way.

It's ironic that something that is a "death art" can help us to get back to a more natural state through the way we move. The most lethal way of moving is also the most natural, and when we move naturally, other things begin to fall into place, to slot in with the giant cogs in the Universe.

With the release of my first book on dim-mak, which contained a brief introduction to the 12 deadly katas, I received many calls and letters from people wanting me to write a separate book and/or video on the "12 secret deadly katas." I thought this would be an easier way, or an introduction into natural movement.

Because we are twentieth-century human beings, we want things unnaturally quicker, and most of us do not wish to spend the time learning a new martial art, especially one as intricate as taijiquan (t'ai chi). The 12 most deadly katas from dim-mak are a way of learning natural circular body movement and can be used alone as a separate martial art.

These 12 katas come from dim-mak and were only given to the most advanced students or family members (those members of a family who inherited the original martial arts systems in China). One technique per year was given over a 12-year period. At the end of that period, the practitioner was so adept at using his hands that no one could match him. It was noted, however, that after such precise training over such a long period, the student did not wish to fight anymore. This is because the movements were invented by people of genius who knew about the flows of *qi* (energy) throughout the body, and these flows would cause a person to become a natural human being again. The person would have the ability to be able to kill with one finger without even thinking about it but, on the other hand, would always find a way not to.

The history of the 12 deadly katas is not clear. However, some, including my main teacher, Chang Yiu-chun, claim that it was Chang San-feng who invented the katas after he had invented dim-mak. Whether the movements of dim-mak (those now known to be taijiquan) or the 12 deadly katas came first is not clear. I tend to think the 12 katas came first, with the movements of taijiquan being a later refinement. Chang became a little paranoid in his older age and did not want others to discover what he had discovered, hence the movements of taijiquan, created to literally cover up the deadly applications and to teach his close students and children.

Chang San-feng was born in 1270 A.D. and probably invented dim-mak and later taijiquan around the beginning of the 1300s, but this also is not absolutely clear. The history is covered in detail in my first book on dim-mak, so I will provide only a nutshell version here.

Chang was an acupuncturist and a martial artist in China. It was his lifetime work to invent the most deadly system of self-defense. So he and a couple of buddies started out by practicing on people, to find out what the acupuncture points did when struck in various directions, with varying pressures, and in different combinations. What they discovered astounded even them, and they decided that it was too dangerous for the general public. Now all we have left is a newer, watered-down version in modern-day t'ai chi—with not many, if any, of the modern masters even knowing the applications of the moves.

The 12 deadly katas were inherited by the Yang family, who kept it secret, only teaching immediate kin. My teacher Chang was one of only three students of Yang Shou-hou, who was the grandson of Yang Lu-ch'an, the founder of the Yang style of taijiquan.

The 12 secret deadly katas teach us many things. The most important is connective body movement. This not only means that every muscle, joint, and bone in the body is interconnected and coordinated but also that the mind is connected to the body, and what the mind says, the body does immediately, with no hesitation. It also teaches economy of movement or, as I call it, "never giving a sucker an even break." So if we are striking with the right palm by turning to the left, we also strike with the left palm as we do this. This is economy of movement at a basic level; the 12 katas take us much further than this. We also learn about subconscious movement. This is where we react to any given situation with the correct movement—without having to think about it. Fa-jing is another area that is taught. Here, we learn how to attack using whole the body, rather than thinking about only the attacking portion of our body. The body explodes, and instantly a palm, fist, or elbow is thrust into this explosion, making for very powerful attacks from very short distances. And we learn about continuous attack, never stopping until the attacker is downed. Each attacking movement is set up by the last, rebounding into the next.

First, we must learn about the solo form or kata. This is not really a continuous kata but 12 separate katas. Later, we have a partner throwing attacks at us. To these we react with one of the 12 different kata techniques, called *san-sau* or *kumite*, moving up and down a training hall, performing each technique on opposite sides.

The 12 deadly katas teach us much, including how to move the body naturally and in tune with the Universe. In this way, we become well physically and then mentally, with body and mind blending as one unit. This is the only way that any good martial art will work against real attacks. The body and mind must act as one, instantly, and the 12 katas are a way to gain this.

All of the following chapters are covered in my video, MTG62, with the same name.

Write to: MTG Publishing, P.O. Box 792, Murwillumbah NSW 2484, Australia. Fax: 011 (61-66) 797028. Ph: 011 (61-66) 797145.

PART ONE

THE SOLO FORMS

The solo forms are an important part of one's training. If we were to train in the two-person method straight away, we would rely upon conditioned responses (those we have learned over the years from incorrect movement taught to us at school or just from rough and tumble in our younger years), and would never learn everything that is to be learned from this method. We must begin at the beginning, learning how to punch all over again, learning how to contract and expand the body so that we become like a huge spring, loading and releasing, in harmony with what the mind is doing and with what is being thrown upon us from an attacker. There is just so much internal work in each kata, which is why it took the students of the old Chinese masters 12 years to learn properly.

Not one part of the body moves without the whole body moving. If we punch to the left, the body turns to the left and causes this punch. Every movement comes from the center and is caused to move by the center's moving. Every part of the body is connected, so that if the center moves, the body moves, right down to the very tips of the fingers. This is *fa-jing*, or "explosive energy."

At first you will find it difficult to gain the power by punching or striking from very short distances. However, as you progress, your mind and body will begin to coordinate and the power will just come. It is always awkward at first to totally change the way we do things, but it comes. I would suggest that you look at one of my videos on this subject so that you can see that this power can be achieved with very little body movement—just a shake from the center is all that is needed.

THE 12 DEADLY PALM TECHNIQUES AND ACUPUNCTURE

We have 12 main acupuncture meridians in our bodies. Each of the 12 deadly katas is related directly to each of these. In turn, each of these techniques or *katas* (forms in Chinese) relates to a different organ in the body, helping to heal anything that could be wrong or is beginning to be wrong with that organ. Each of the katas also relates to a different element. For instance, the first kata relates to fire, or the heart. This kata helps in the healing of the heart and also helps to dispel any condition that has to do with too much water, etc. There is even a correct time of day for each kata to be performed. This is not that important, although for the kata to be at its best where healing is concerned, it is advisable to do it at that particular time. It does not matter what time you do the katas when only the self-defense applications are concerned. I will be giving the healing applications as I cover each kata. Note that all of the acupuncture or dim-mak points and their locations are covered in great detail in both of my previous books, *Dim-Mak: Death Point Striking* and *Advanced Dim-Mak: The Finer Points of Death-Point Striking*, both published by Paladin Press. If you are not familiar with the points and their locations, these two books will provide the background you will need to gain the most from this book.

QIGONG

Before beginning each of the 12 katas, a *qigong* or breathing technique specific to the particular kata is performed. This "sets up" the whole kata so you will not only make it a physical movement but take each of the techniques into the internal and so that it will be good for health. Each qigong causes different qi flows to happen in the body, and this flow is specific to what you are about to do in the self-defense area. The qigong is not only good for health but also helps in gaining the fa-jing power necessary for the specific technique. The qigong concentrates the qi into the palms and is also very good for health.

CHAPTER 1

SOLO KATA #1

Snake Hands

This kata derives its name from the way the hands move, in an "S" shape, or what most people think a snake looks like when it is standing up ready to strike.

HEALING

The first of the 12 katas is associated with the heart. Its element is fire, and for the healing to be at its greatest, it should be done between the hours of 11 A.M. and 1 P.M. Being associated with the heart, this kata naturally works upon the blood vessels. It will have a great healing effect upon the heart and blood vessels, even if you do not do it at the prescribed time. Its effect is just greater at the correct time.

NOTE: Although each of the 12 katas has its own specific qigong, the whole kata may be done slowly, as one would perform a taiji kata or form. Doing the kata in this way, we gain the qigong benefits described in each of the chapters on the solo katas under the qigong section.

THE QIGONG

The opening stance for the snake hands kata, or the first form, is also your first qigong.

Please note that in the qigong part of these exercises, we breathe in and out through the nose. However, when we begin the self-defense part of the katas, we breathe in through the nose and exhale explosively through the mouth, making a noise that is representative of the particular attack—usually a "pah!" type of sound and never a more flowing "hah!" type of sound.

The first qigong calms the heart and spirit so that the whole being will be relaxed, or in a state of *sung*. Sung is when the body moves without the physical mind knowing it has moved, like when you are just falling off to sleep, perhaps thinking about a technique, and all of a sudden your fist is thrown upward at great speed and power, it wakes you and you don't know what has happened. When you

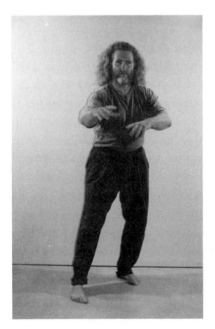

Figure 1

try to recreate this consciously, you are unable to. When the mind, "thinks" about a technique, time is taken in this conscious thought, whereas, if the movement is done without the conscious mind interacting, then tremendous speed and power are achieved. Some like to call this supernatural power, but it is quite natural.

Stand relaxed with one foot (the right one first) in front of the other. Don't make it a large open stance, but rather a more mobile stance, with the feet about shoulder width apart. The feet are almost parallel to each other, and the weight is distributed more onto the rear foot. The hands are held loosely in front, with the right hand slightly in front of the left (the same as the feet). The right palm is held palm slightly downward, as is the left (fig. 1). Your shoulders are relaxed and rounded, the tongue is held naturally with the tip lightly pressed to the upper palate just behind the ridge of the teeth, and the breathing is deep, relaxed, and not forced. You imagine a force moving up the backbone from the sacrum on each inhalation and over the head down to the point in between the eyes. Then, on the exhalation, you imagine that same force flowing down the back of your tongue to a point inside your body about 3 inches below your navel (the *tantien*). Stand like this for about three minutes, relaxing every portion of your body. Become more relaxed upon each exhalation.

Now you begin to breathe out of your palms on each exhalation. Still imagine that force coming up your backbone, but now, on the exhalation, send the force out of your palms from a point called *Laogung* (Palace of Labor), or Pericardium 8 (fig. 2). As you do this, you will feel a warmth around the point, which indicates that the qi is indeed being sent out of this point.

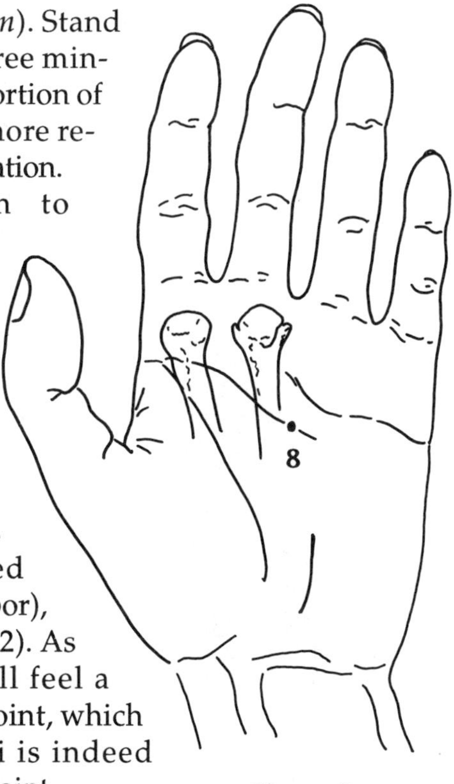

Figure 2

Laogung is the point where the qi emanates from, either for the healing or for the killing. Close your fist, and where the longest finger touches on the inside of your palm, this is the point. By simply looking at this point and "breathing" out of it, you will cause a redness to occur all over the palm (motley skin), which will concentrate around the point. Look at the point, and when you exhale, imagine that the breath is traveling out of it. The breath, of course, doesn't actually go out from that point, but by visualizing this, you cause the qi to travel out of it. Breathe out of Laogung for another minute. This is the qigong of the first kata. You must also do this qigong on the other side, i.e., you reverse the palms and feet.

Over the course of many years of teaching, I have worked out a way to show the internal movements, those that are normally too small to see from the outside. I simply exaggerate the movements so that they can be seen and then take them smaller and smaller until they cannot be seen. That's how I will attempt to show the small movements in this book. Please note that I will be numbering the exaggerated photos as EX fig. 3 or EX fig. 4 to indicate that what is shown is not the way the movement is to be done but rather an exaggeration of what it should look like. I will also be showing the real movements in photos next to the exaggerated movements. Also note that many of the photos will not need to have an exaggerated photo to back them up.

THE KATA

The first of the 12 katas involves the use of two fists and two palms in retaliation to a straight punch to our face. (You will be defending yourself against actual punches when you learn how to do the katas in a kumite, or fighting way, in Chapter 13.)

From the beginning posture, your body twists from

the waist slightly to your left, moving your upper body over slightly to your right, and spirals from the waist in a counterclockwise direction. This will begin to push out your right palm, which has begun to turn over from its initial palm-down position. As you begin this movement, you will begin to breathe in. Remember that this whole technique, when learned, will only take a split second to execute, so the breathing will not be coordinated until you have it down to this speed. In fact, it is not fast at all; it is explosive, or fa-jing. There is a quick inhalation on this movement, followed by an exhalation on the rest of the technique (fig. 3) and (EX fig. 4)

Notice that the body has been compressed at the right-hand side of the waist. The body is now like a spring, wound up and ready to release.

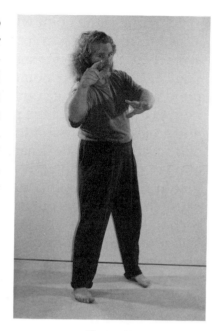

Figure 3

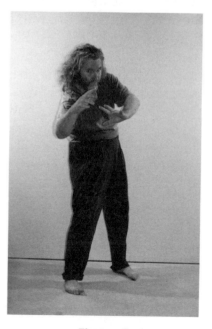

Figure 4

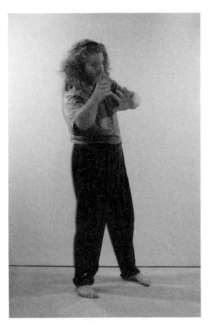

The waist now turns further to your left as your hips begin to "open up" or release the spring. Your right palm has turned over more at about a 45-degree angle to the ground (fig. 5 and EX fig. 6).

Figure 5

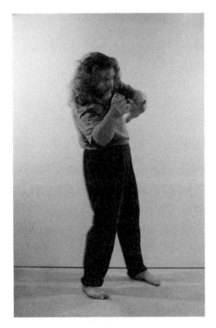

Figure 6

Your waist reaches its fullest turn to your left and is just about to begin its turn back to the right when your right palm turns fully over to palm upward and the fist closes (upon impact). This causes the fist to rotate in a lateral counterclockwise direction (fig. 7). Notice that the fist is held in the "tiger paw" (fig. 8) with the longest (middle) finger's knuckle protruding. This is the striking part.

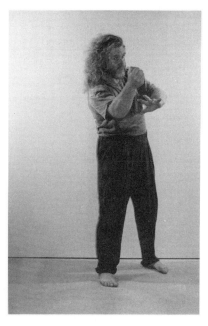

Figure 7

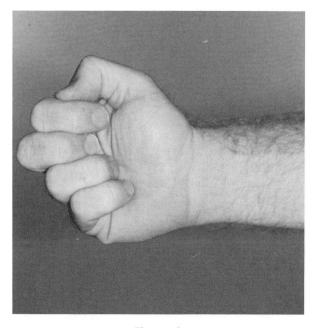

Figure 8

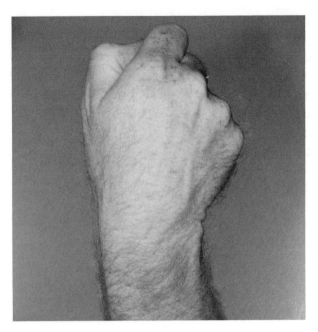

Figure 9

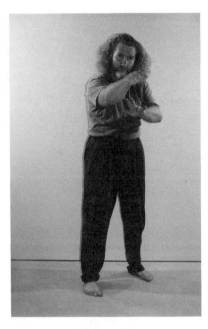

Figure 10

Your waist now explodes back to your right, taking the power from the initial explosive turning to your left. As you do this, your right fist continues the circular movement back over to your right. Notice how the fist is held with relation to the wrist (fig. 9). The tiger paw knuckle is now withdrawn, and contact will be made with the last two knuckles of the ring finger and small finger (fig. 10).

The waist now turns fully to the right, and as it begins to turn to the left again, the right fist makes contact (fig. 11).

As your waist is turning fully to the left again, your right foot takes a small step forward and both of your elbows open up slightly. The right side of your abdomen is now contracted (fig. 12 and EX fig. 13). You have also changed your right fist into an open palm. The waist is now "sprung" again ready to release for the final blow.

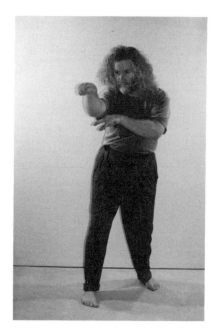

Figure 11

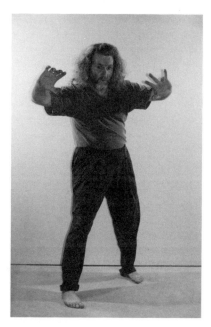

Figure 12

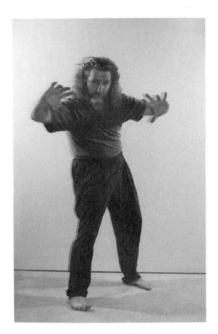

Figure 13

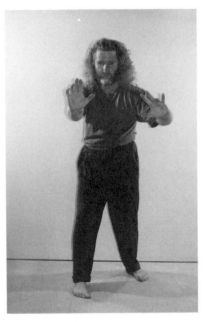

Figure 14

As your waist turns back to the right, you release the spring tension in your waist and strike with your right palm, squeezing in your elbow to give a clockwise twist to your palm as it strikes (fig. 14). Your waist has turned back to the right and is now beginning to turn back to the left. As it does, your left palm also with the aid of the left elbow squeezing inward, strikes lower with a twisting counterclockwise strike (fig. 15). The waist now flicks back to the right and center position (fig. 16).

It seems like there is a lot of turning of the waist, and people wonder how to get in all of these turns in a split second. But when you see this done, it seems as if the whole body has just shook violently. It is almost impossible to actually see these movements they are so explosive.

You can see from the above why it took a

whole year to learn properly. I could have just said to throw a punch, then throw a circular punch and two palm strikes, but this would be as much to dim-mak and fa-jing and mind/body coordination as a snail is to a Porsche!

The main area is the waist, as this is what causes fa-jing. If the waist is stiff, then fa-jing is not possible. This is why taiji devotes so much time to getting a loose waist.

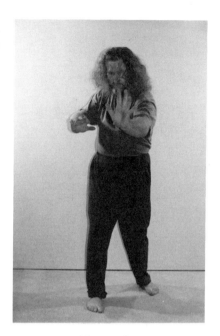

Figure 15

The first fist should literally snap like a whip; you should actually hear the snap. The power is in the waist; if you are not getting it, work on the waist (or get the video).

An Exercise to Gain a Loose Waist

Stand opposite your partner with feet parallel and shoulder width apart. You tell yourself that you are trying to distinguish between "waist" and "hip." The

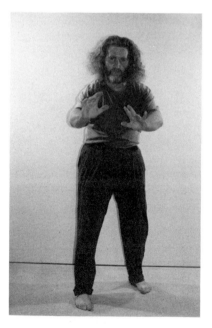

Figure 16

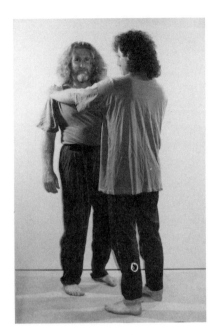

Figure 17

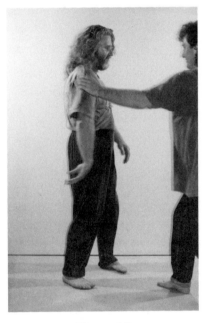

Figure 18

sacrum (that big, flat bone at the bottom of your backbone, just above your coccyx, or tailbone) and that which is below it is the hip. That which is above the sacrum is the waist. You try to hold your hips facing your partner; they do not move. You loosen your waist so that your partner is able to turn your shoulders by pushing on one hand and pulling with the other (fig. 17). Your partner must tell you if you are either helping him to turn your waist or using your muscle pressure to stop him. Both are wrong. The waist is normally hard to turn and will require some work by your partner. When your partner lets go of your shoulders suddenly, your waist should spring back to the front a little too much, so that the shoulders will rock back and forth for a couple of free swings before returning to center. This is a loose waist.

Your partner will have to jump back out of the way if your waist is loose, as your arms will spring outward by the centrifugal force and strike him in the crown jewels. However, if you are "helping" by turning your own waist, then when he lets go, your shoulders will just stay there and won't spring back. If you are pushing against him, then he won't be able to let your shoulders go, as they will follow him too quickly. Figure 18 shows the swing after he lets go.

You should practice the first kata over and over until you are able to do the whole technique on the count of one.

The next part is to learn the whole technique on the reverse side. You stand with your left foot and hand forward and do the whole thing again. Do this until you have both sides down to a "one" count. When you have this down, you will not even wait when you change steps, but rather you will do one side, then as you take a step forward you will already be doing the first punch. This is the way you will be doing it with a partner later as well.

CHAPTER 2

SOLO KATA 2
Straight Hands

The beginning posture of this solo form is, again, its specific qigong posture.

Like all of the beginning qigong postures, this one causes great calmness and internal/external stability. It can be used, for instance, when one is going for a job interview or is about to take an exam, for this qigong is the attacking qigong. It gives us the necessary mind/body energy or qi to go forth and attack whatever it is that we have to do. In the basic and purely martial arts application, this attacking qi will be used against an attacker. But the qi is used the same way, whether in a job interview or a physical attack.

HEALING

This kata works upon the small intestine as well as the blood vessels, and its element in Chinese traditional medicine (CTM) is fire. Its time of day is between the hours of 1 P.M. and 3 P.M.

THE QIGONG

Again, you stand with one foot slightly forward of the other. This time I will begin with the left foot forward. The left hand is held at about shoulder height, while the right palm is held lower, about stomach height. Again, the whole body is in a state of sung, with only the right muscles being used to hold the arms in this position. The tongue is again just touching the upper teeth ridge, and the whole posture is the same as for the qigong for Snake Hands, or Solo Kata No. 1.

There is a difference, though. It is in the way we are thinking. Upon the inhalation, imagine that as the lower abdomen expands, it is filling up with qi, flowing up through your feet from a point called Kidney 1 (fig. 19). The qi flows up through the legs and into the cavity caused by the expanding abdomen. Concentrate more on the lower abdomen rather than the upper chest area, and do not fill out your chest at all (fig. 20).

As you breathe out (of your nose), imagine that the breath, or qi, is rushing out of your left fingers as they are stretched a little (open them). The torso squashes or contracts on your left-hand side as you do this (fig. 21 and EX fig. 22).

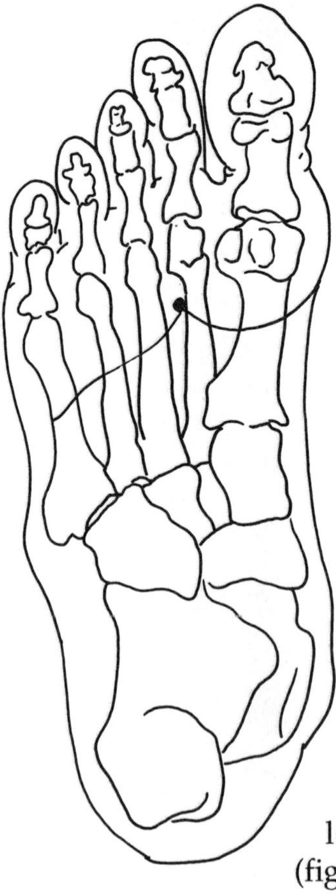

Figure 19

22

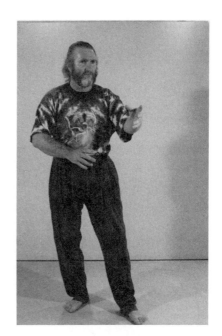

Figure 20

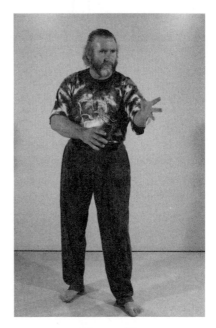

Figure 21

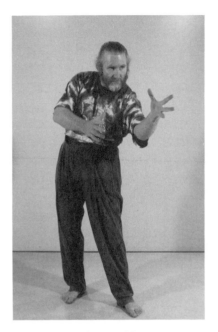

Figure 22

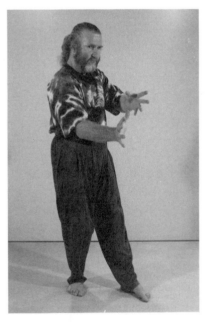

Figure 23

However, do not exhale all of your breath. Only half of the exhalation should happen while stretching your left fingers and so on. On the other half of the exhalation, the left fingers relax again while the right-hand side of the abdomen contracts and twists slightly to your left and your right palm flexes (yang) and is pushed slightly forward. Now imagine that the second half of your exhalation is being pumped out of your right palm's Laogung point (fig. 23 and EX fig. 24). As you finish, ready to breathe in again, your palms and body relax, returning to the starting posture, ready to inhale again, filling up the lower abdomen. You should not force your breath, as this will cause tension and high blood pressure, but rather just inhale and exhale as normal, relaxed. The movements should adjust to the breath. Do not adjust the breath to the movement. You do 10 rounds of this qigong and then do the whole 10 on the reverse side. Then reverse your stance again, ready to begin the kata.

Upon finishing your tenth round of the above qigong exercise, and having already begun the eleventh by breathing in, you have four strikes to execute upon the exhalation.

THE KATA

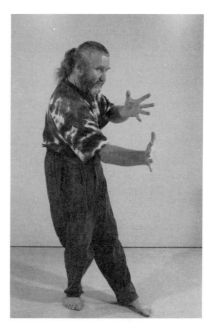

Figure 24

Take half a step to the front with your left foot as your left fingers jab forward, while turning your waist slightly to your right. The fingers stretch slightly (fig. 25). As the waist turns to the left, your right palm now strikes forward and flexes as your left fingers relax (fig. 26).

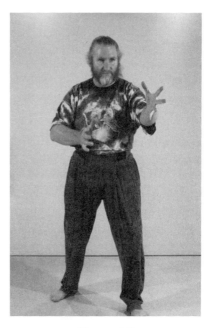

Figure 25

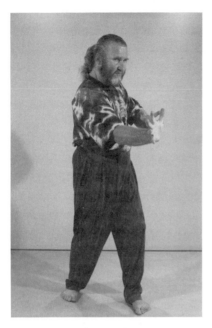

Figure 26

Rebounding from the previous turn, your waist does a slight turn to your right as your right palm relaxes (fig. 27). Your waist turns to the left and your right "penetration" punch is thrown out, snapping over so that the small finger is on top. The striking part here are the two largest knuckles of the fist. This punch will be dealt with later when I show how to put it all together with a partner (fig. 28).

The right fist does not swing out but is thrown straight forward. It has the appearance of a slightly round punch because it snaps over upon impact. The left palm also attacks with a shake outward as the right fist attacks. It's as if it is hitting an arm away. It gets its power from the whole fa-jing shake, made for the whole body. This is the beauty of fa-jing—all one has to do is shake the whole body and put the correct attacking

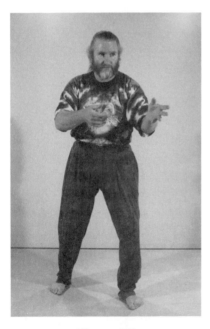

Figure 27

portions of the body into the correct position. The body does the work, not the individual peripherals.

The rebound from this attack leads into the next movement. The waist is coiled, ready to strike as the left foot is brought back level with the right foot. The right fist (held loosely) is brought back slightly, ready to attack again while the left hand is held in an on-guard position (fig. 29 and EX fig. 30).

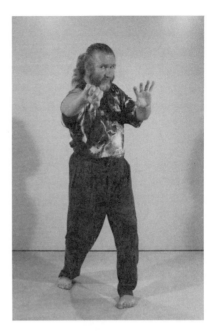

Figure 28

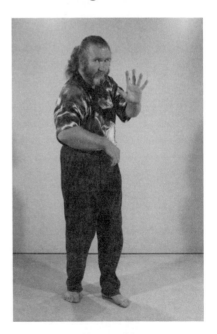

Figure 29

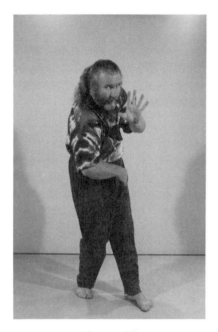

Figure 30

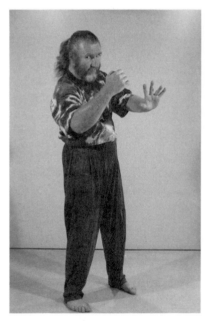

Figure 31

The right foot steps forward and the waist snaps to your right, thus thrusting out your right backfist (fig. 31). The left palm again does a small strike outward, gaining its power from the fajing shake. The waist now rebounds back to your left and your right wrist is jerked backward, thus flicking out the back of your fist (fig. 32). The rebound from this attack turns your waist to your right as your right wrist is cocked ready, held in a yin shape (relaxed). Your waist now turns violently to your left, which causes your right palm to be thrust forward and in an arc from right to left (fig. 33). Again, the left palm also strikes out to the left slightly just before the right palm makes contact. (I say "makes contact," although no contact has been made at this stage, as we are only doing the solo kata. Later, when I show the two-person kata, you will see why you are doing these move-ments.)

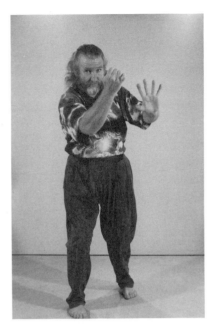

Figure 32

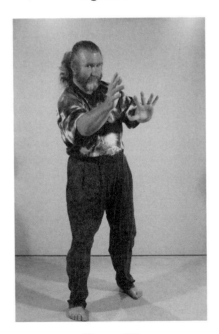

Figure 33

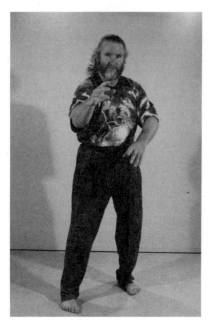

The waist now returns to center position as your right palm relaxes (fig. 34). You are now in the opposite position from which you began this second kata and can perform the whole technique on the opposite side.

Learn this kata fully on the one side first. Then do it on the opposite side, beginning with your right foot forward. Learn slowly at first, then try to feel the fa-jing of the body. Shake the hips and waist and simply throw out a loose fist as you do this. Do not force your fist; just let it go, and if hips and waist are doing the right thing, then you will begin to feel the great power of fa-jing.

Figure 34

CHAPTER 3

SOLO KATA #3

Changing Hand

This is the first technique where only the palm is used. It is called Changing Hand because the palm changes explosively to attack using different parts of the palm.

The specific qigong associated with this palm is also its starting posture. This qigong imparts the ability to change, not only in the self-defense area but also in life. It is used when one is "in a rut," for instance. It is said to cause energies of change within the body to come alive. In the self-defense area, it enables us to change to varying situations and attacks and to use the right tool for the right situation subconsciously.

HEALING

This kata works upon the kidneys and it governs the bone marrow. Its time of day is between the hours of 5 P.M. and 7 P.M. Its element in CTM is water.

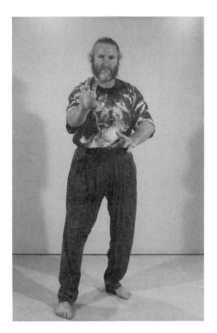

Figure 35

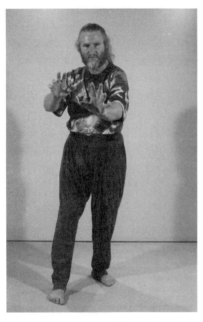

Figure 36

THE QIGONG

The basic body positioning is the same as the first posture with regard to the sung state, the positioning of the tongue, the relaxing shoulders, and so on covered in the first chapter. This will remain the same for the 12 qigongs.

With the right foot forward, hold the right palm like a claw. Hold the left palm with the fingers pointing away from you (fig. 35).

Again, coordinate the breath with the movement. As you inhale through your nose, your waist turns slightly to your right, which thrusts your left fingers forward. The palm stretches slightly as you do this (fig. 36). Be sure not to turn your hips; they must remain pointing to the front. Only the waist turns. As you exhale, your waist turns slightly to your left, which thrusts out your slightly flexed right palm (fig. 37).

Repeat this whole exercise 10 times. Imagine that you are breathing in through the tips of your left fingers and then take the breath out through your right Laogung point. That point will become slightly red in color when you do this correctly. You do the whole round 10 times on both sides, then reverse the final stance so that you are ready to begin the kata.

THE KATA

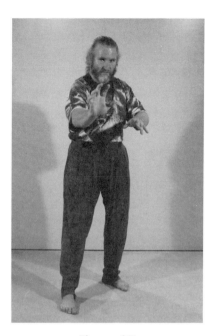

Figure 37

Upon finishing the tenth round and taking the next inhalation, step forward with your right foot and thrust your left fingers forward while turning your waist slightly to the right (fig. 38). As you breathe out, thrust your right "claw" forward and turn your waist to your left (fig. 39). The waist turns slightly to your right again as your right palm drops and turns over (fig. 40). Turn your waist to your left as the

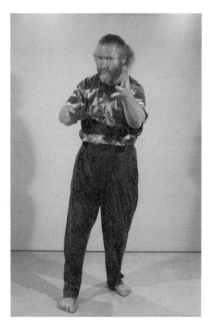

Figure 38

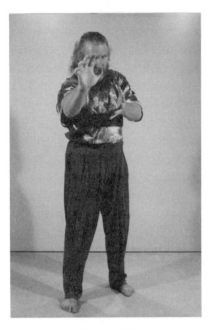

Figure 39

back of your right palm slaps forward in a slightly downward motion and your waist turns back to the right upon impact. This is not unlike the backfist you did in the second kata, whipping your arm back to gain the power (fig. 41).

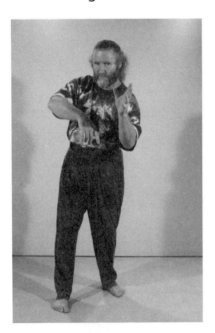

Figure 40

You draw your right palm back as your waist turns to the right (fig. 42).

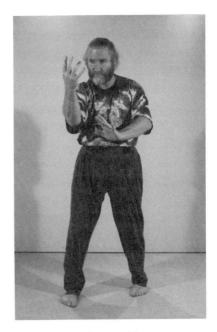

Figure 41

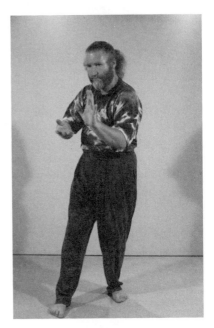

Figure 42

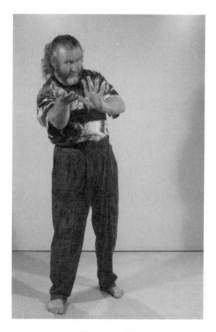

Figure 43

Your waist now turns to the left as your right fingers jab forward (fig. 43). All of this time (only a very short time), the left palm has just stayed where it is and has moved accordingly with the motion of the body.

As your waist turns to your right, your right palm makes like it is stabbing something as your right foot comes back to being even with your left foot (fig. 44). Your left foot steps forward as your upward-facing left palm strikes (fig. 45). The movement of your right palm is in accordance with what your left palm is doing, i.e., it is doing the opposite—jerking backward.

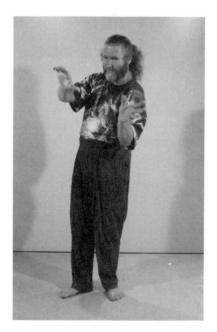

Figure 44

The whole routine has only taken around a second to execute, but take it easy at first—don't worry if you can't get it all done on the one exhalation. And, again, the waist has only gone back and forth a few times. Doing it slowly, we think that the waist is doing a lot of movement, but seeing it done, it looks as if the waist has just shaken violently.

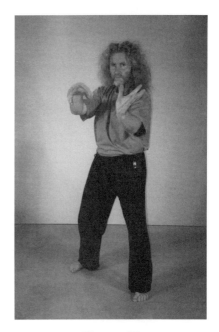

Figure 45

You end up with your left foot forward in the right position to do this whole routine on the reverse side.

Do this on both sides any number of times, perhaps working your way up and down the dojo.

Your right palm is held relaxed in front at about chest height (fig. 47). The body positioning is the same as for all of the qigongs (covered in the first kata).

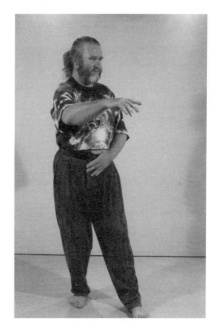

Figure 47

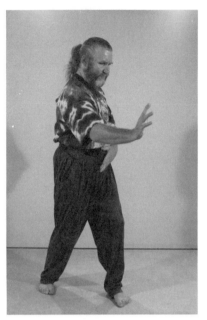

On the exhalation, you turn your waist to your left and compress the right side of your abdomen as your right palm flexes slightly, going with the movement and moving to your left naturally (fig. 48 and EX fig. 49). Your left palm presses slightly inward at the tantien point.

Figure 48

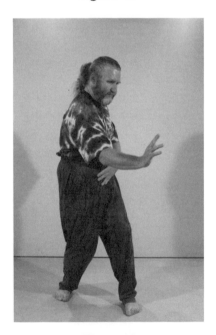

Figure 49

DIM-MAK'S 12 MOST DEADLY KATAS

Your waist now turns to your right and the abdomen is compressed on your left side as your right palm is lifted naturally out to your right with that movement. The palm relaxes to a yin shape with the movement (fig. 50 and EX fig. 51). This is done on the inhalation, and your left palm relaxes the pushing inward that it did for the exhalation.

This qigong will not work if all of the basic posturing is not adhered to, such as the relaxation of the entire body, slightly closed eyes, and so on.

With this qigong, you imagine that the breath is coming in through Laogung on your right palm and going into the Laogung point in your left palm (the one that is placed on your abdomen). On the exhalation, you imagine that the breath is going from the left Laogung and out into infinity through the right Laogung.

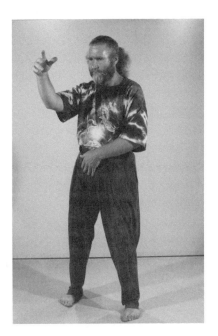

Figure 50

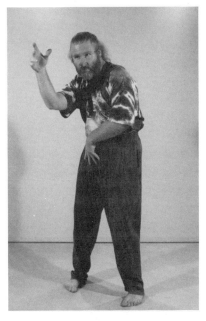

Figure 51

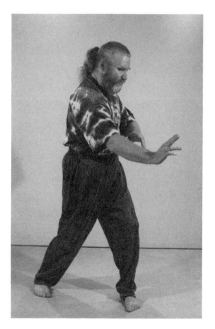

Figure 52

You perform the above qigong 10 times on both sides, then reverse your stance to be in the right-handed stance for the beginning of the kata.

THE KATA

Take a half step out to your left diagonally with your left foot. As you do this, your right palm is thrust downward and to your left in a yang shape. The left palm is in a yin shape, ready to move, as in Figure 52. The right palm bends and, with the slight turning of your waist to your right, is pulled to your right as your left palm strikes upward with its knife edge (fig. 53). In Figure 54, the left palm bends and pulls over to your left with the turning of your waist to your left. The knife edge of your right palm slams downward to your left as you bring your weight onto your left foot (fig. 55). You now take a step

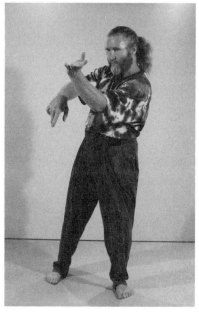

Figure 53

forward with your right foot and repeat the whole procedure on the reverse side.

Once you have learned this slowly, you must speed up the whole kata so that it is the waist that is initiating all of the movement. The palms only move up and down; it is the waist that gives the movement the lateral motion.

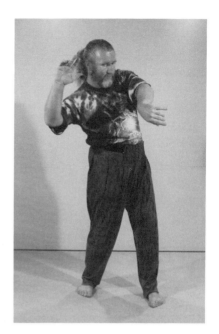

Figure 54

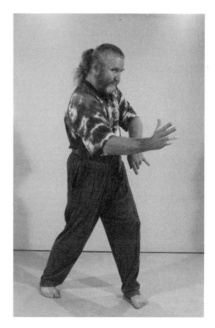

Figure 55

CHAPTER 5

SOLO KATA 5
Waving Hand

This kata is called Waving Hand because of the way that the palm shakes upon impact. It makes use of the palm, the fingers, the tiger paw fist, and the elbow.

The qigong for this one is again its beginning stance, and this qigong works upon the head, making for much better concentration. In the martial sense, it results in greater coordination between brain and hands.

HEALING

The internal organ that this kata works upon is the Pericardium, the sack that protects the heart, and it is also associated with the blood vessels. Its element in Chinese medicine is fire, and its time of day is between the hours of 7 P.M. and 9 P.M.

THE QIGONG

Stand with your right foot forward. Your right palm is held as if ready to strike something with the tips of the fingers. The left palm is lightly touching the outside

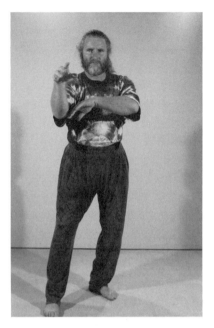

Figure 56

of the right forearm. You are in a state of sung, and your qi is concentrated in your lower abdomen. Your tongue is touching the upper palate as for all of the qigongs (fig. 56). As you inhale, your waist turns to your right and your right wrist becomes yin. As you turn, the fingers of your left palm slide down the outside of your right forearm. It is important that your eyes are focused directly ahead of you. You might like to put something on the wall to concentrate upon. Although your waist is turning, your eyes still look forward, i.e., you are looking out of the corners of the eyes. There is a slight compression on the left side of your abdomen (fig. 57 and EX fig. 58).

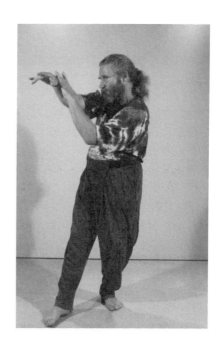

Figure 57

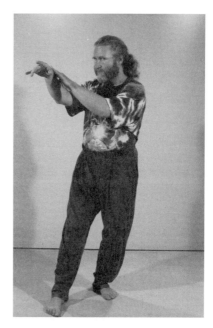

Figure 58

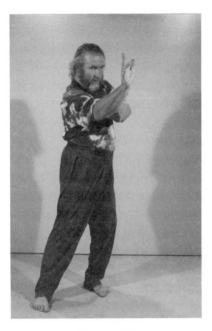

Figure 59

As you exhale, the waist turns to the left, the right wrist flexes, and the fingers of the left palm are rubbed up the inside of your right forearm. Again, the focus is straight ahead. The eyes do not move as the body turns, so you must actually look out of the corners of your eyes (fig. 59).

As your waist turns back to the right, your left palm again rubs down the outside of your right forearm and you perform the whole qigong again. Do this also starting with the left foot forward and the hands reversed. Do this qigong 10 times on both sides. At the finish of the tenth time on the left side, you again reverse your footwork to begin the kata.

THE KATA

With your right foot forward, you have inhaled and have turned your waist to your right and rubbed the outside of your right arm downward with your left fingers. (This was the beginning of the qigong).

Place some weight onto the right foot as your waist turns to your left. Your left hand is thrust outward to your left as your right fingers are thrust forward (fig. 60). Your weight shifts back onto your left foot again, and your waist turns back to your right as you rebound from the previous movement. Your right palm has turned over and is beginning to form a tiger fist. Your left palm has also come back (fig. 61).

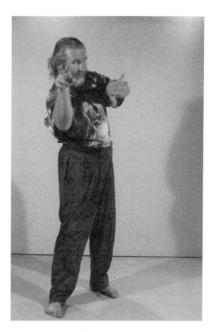

Figure 60

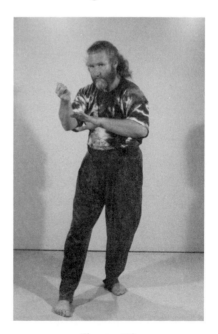

Figure 61

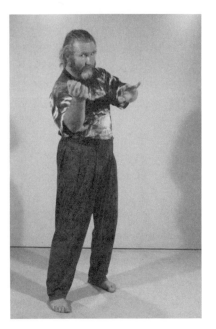

Rebounding from the first strike, your right tiger paw fist snaps forward as your left palm again strikes out to your left. Your waist first turns to the left, and as your right fist strikes, it snaps back to your right, making it a fa-jing move (figs. 62 and 63).

Figure 62

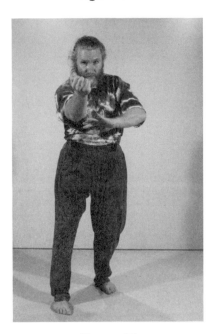

Figure 63

Rebounding from the last strike, you take a step to your left with your left foot forward slightly, as you slam your right palm downward. The right side of your abdomen is compressed, loading like a spring, and your waist has turned slightly to your left (fig. 64).

Continuing, your right palm makes like it is grabbing something. As your waist turns to your right, your right palm pulls. Using the power of the waist, the left palm strikes forward, using the knife edge with the palm facing upward (fig. 65).

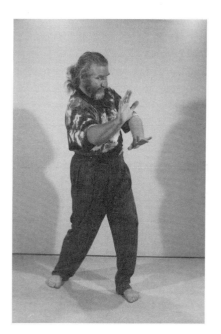

Figure 64

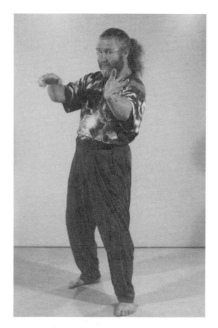

Figure 65

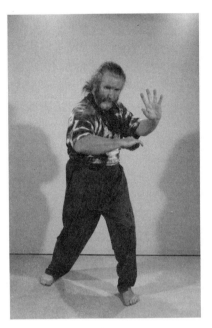

Figure 66

Still using the last fa-jing movement, as your waist rebounds back to your left, you utilize this power by striking outward to your left with your left palm and striking forward with your right elbow (fig. 66).

You have performed two fa-jing shakes here. The first two moves were on the first fa-jing shake, while the last two were on the second. The step with the left foot and the strike downward was a movement all by itself. You end up with your left foot forward to begin again on the other side with the left palm forward.

CHAPTER 6

SOLO KATA #6
Breaking Hand

The beginning posture of this kata is the specific qigong for this kata. This qigong builds up the fire in the tantien. It provides us with more qi to be able to work with in the martial sense.

On a day-to-day level, this qigong will help in overcoming tight situations, such as dealing with a new boss, going for a tough job interview, and so on. But be warned—it can result in too much qi circulating, and your potential employer might think you are too positive! It is a good idea to combine this qigong with the No. 1 qigong, which knocks off the harsh edges that you get by doing this one. Martially, we need this hard energy, and we even need it in our daily lives, but sometimes it can be a little too great.

HEALING

This kata works upon the Sanjiao meridian, or the Triple Warmer meridian. This means that it basically works upon the whole body. We have three "heating" spaces in our body that do work for us: the lower heater (warmer), the middle heater, and the upper heater. The lower heater deals with elimination, while the middle warmer deals with digestion and the upper warmer deals with the brain, respiration, etc. This kata's time of day is between the hours of 9 P.M. and 11 P.M. The part of the body it controls are the blood vessels, while its Chinese medicine element is fire.

THE QIGONG

This time you will be inhaling through the nose and exhaling through the mouth.

Stand with your right foot forward. The whole body is again in a state of sung. The tongue is resting on the upper palate and the breathing is deep but not forced. The palms are allowed to just hang there. The right one is held thumb up and fingers pointing away, while the left is held with palm pointing away (fig. 67).

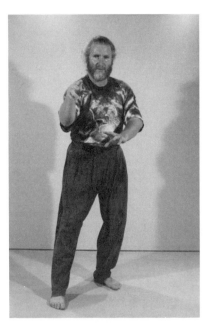

As you inhale through your nose, you turn your waist to your left, which brings both palms to your left. (The palms have not actually moved independently of the body, but rather the body has moved them.) A small amount of weight has shifted to your right foot, but not more than 40 percent (fig. 68).

As you begin to exhale, all of your weight is shifted back onto your left foot, while your right palm

Figure 67

bends, as if pulling. Your waist is beginning to turn back to your right. Your left palm is being thrust out over the top of your right palm (fig. 69). As you turn to your right and sit back fully onto your left foot, your left palm is thrust out to your left, while your right palm is kept in line with your center as you exhale completely out of your mouth with the tongue on the lower palate just touching the lower teeth ridge. This causes a "ha" sound.

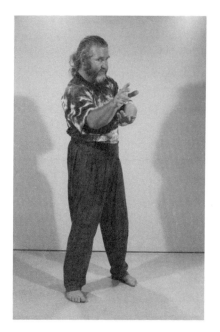

Figure 68

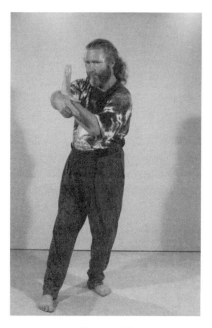

Figure 69

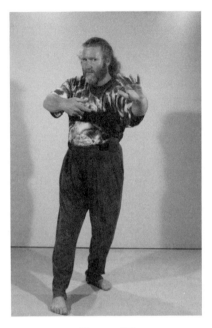

Figure 70

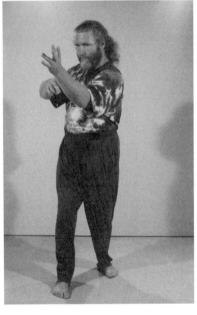

Figure 71

Although your head has turned to the right with your waist, your eyes have stayed with your left palm, i.e., you are looking out of the corners of your eyes to the left (fig. 70).

You must now perform the hand movements in reverse, but do not change the footing just yet. This is still part of the first round. You bring your left palm over to your right as you inhale and transfer no more than 40 percent of your weight to your right foot (fig. 71). The tongue is back up on the upper palate. As you exhale, your tongue again goes down onto the lower palate as you turn your waist to your left. Your left palm now acts as if pulling, while your right palm is beginning to be thrust out to your right (fig. 72). Your weight is beginning to shift back onto your left foot.

As you exhale fully through your mouth, you turn your waist to your left and extend your right palm outward as your left palm stays positioned in your center. You are looking out of the corners of your eyes to the right, focusing on your right palm (fig. 73).

You are now able to repeat from the beginning, as this has been one round. Do it 10 times and then return to the beginning posture, reverse the stance, and do it another 10 times, changing the stance at the end so that you can begin the kata with the right foot forward.

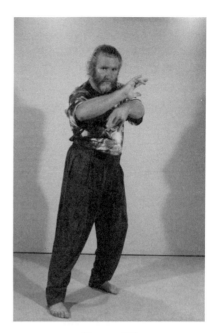

Figure 72

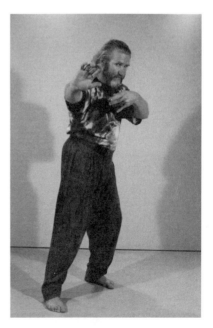

Figure 73

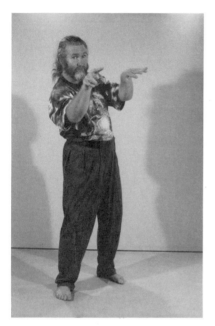

Figure 74

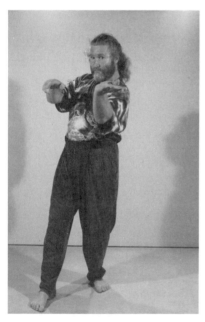

Figure 75

THE KATA

With the right foot forward, you do exactly the same beginning move as in Solo Kata No. 5. The left palm is thrust out to your left as your waist turns to your left and your right palm makes like it is poking something with the tips of the fingers (fig. 74). Your weight has shifted slightly onto your right foot but no more than 40 percent.

With the rebound of the first move and as your waist turns back to your right, your left palm thrusts forward as your right palm makes like it is grabbing and pulling something, using the power of the waist only. The weight has moved back onto the left foot, and your waist has turned to your right (fig. 75).

The waist now turns back to your left as a slight amount of weight is placed onto the right foot. The left palm is thrust out to your left,

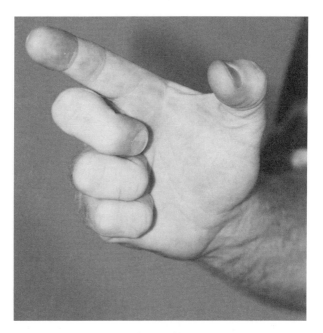

Figure 76

while the right palm is thrust forward and held as in Figure 76. The whole body is held as in Figure 77.

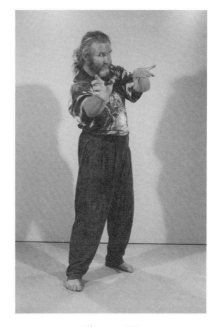

Figure 77

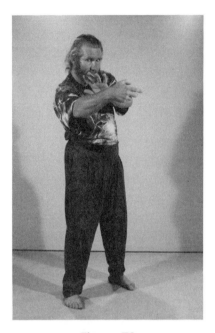

Figure 78

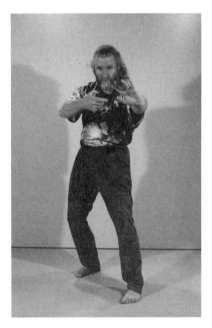

Figure 79

With the weight still slightly forward, you turn your waist to your left as your right palm bends. Your left palm does not move because the body has turned to the left, bringing the left palm in line with the center (fig. 78). As you sit back onto your left leg and the waist turns to your right, the right palm pulls in toward your center as the left palm is thrust forward over the top of your right palm. As you pull your right palm back, your right foot also retreats to no more than the left foot. As your left palm is thrust forward, your left foot comes forward. This is called a "change step." The front foot comes back before the back foot goes to the forward position (fig. 79). You are now in the opposite position, able to do the whole round on the reverse side.

Remember, as I am talking you through these katas, that although it may sound like a long time, the last kata, for instance, takes only a fraction of a second to do. But build up the speed slowly.

CHAPTER 7

SOLO KATA 7
Willow Hand

The beginning posture is again the particular qigong for this kata, called Willow Hand because of the way the palms move like the branches of the willow tree in a breeze, back and forth.

This qigong allows for the swapping of the different energies in the body. It causes you to be able to change rapidly, not only in the self-defense area, but also in your daily life.

HEALING

The time of day for this kata is between the hours of 11 P.M. and 1 A.M. This is a very important kata, as it works upon the gall bladder and controls the muscles and sinews. The specific Gall Bladder point that has a great effect upon the muscles and sinews is GB 34, located just below the knee over that big lump on the outside of the leg (fig. 80). Used in acupuncture, it heals any problems to do with the muscles and sinews. Used in dim-mak, it damages the muscles and sinews, in particular, those of the leg. Its Chinese traditional medicine element is wood.

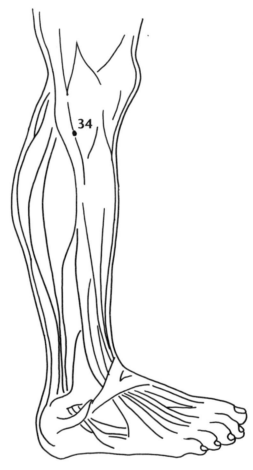

Figure 80

THE QIGONG

With the left foot forward, hold the left palm forward of the right, which is held in a little, closed fist (fig. 81). The breathing is all through the nose this time, and the tongue is touching the upper palate. The body is in a state of sung.

As you inhale, begin to move your weight onto your left foot. Your left palm is withdrawn to under your right elbow, while the right fist rises to upper chest height. The waist has turned to your left (fig. 82). The next four moves are performed as you exhale.

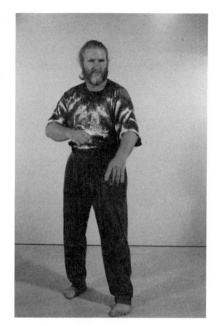

Figure 81

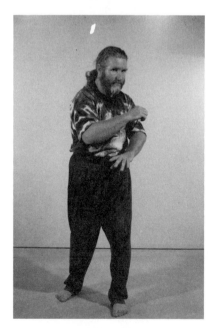

Figure 82

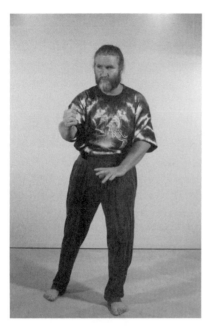

Turn your waist to your right as the back of your right fist is thrust out to your right. You are beginning to exhale (fig. 83). Continuing the exhalation, turn your waist back to your left as your left palm is now thrust forward, and your right palm is withdrawn. Your weight begins to shift back onto the rear foot (fig. 84).

Figure 83

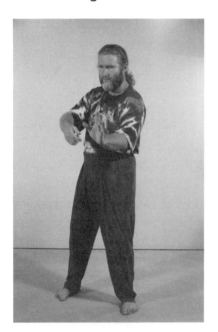

Figure 84

Continuing exhalation and the moving back onto the rear foot, withdraw the left palm as you thrust the right palm forward. Your waist has turned to the left (fig. 85). Your weight is now on the rear foot.

Complete the exhalation as you turn your waist to your right and hook your right palm, pulling it inward as your left palm is thrust outward (fig. 86).

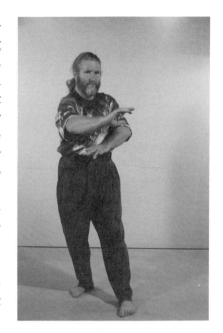

Figure 85

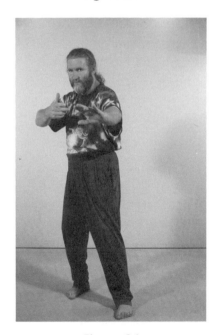

Figure 86

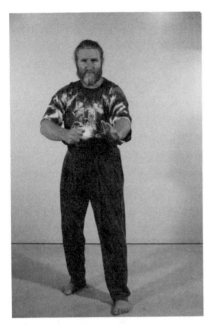

Figure 87

Breathe in as you turn your waist back to center and place your palms in the beginning position, ready to do this qigong again (fig. 87). Repeat the whole round by six times on this side and then take a step forward to repeat the whole thing six times on the reverse side. Take another step forward so that your left foot is leading again for the beginning of the kata.

THE KATA

From the beginning qigong posture with left foot forward, step out to your left diagonally with the left foot. As you step, the right fist is drawn up your center and "loaded," ready to strike. The left palm has come under the right elbow (fig. 88). You place your weight onto the left foot and attack with the right backfist out to your right. Your left wrist stays at your center and

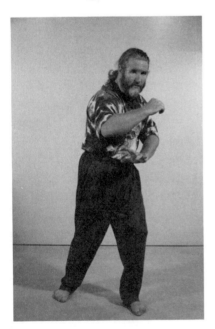

Figure 88

the waist is aligned to where your hips are pointing, out to your left diagonally (fig. 89).

Stay weighted on the left foot as your right palm hooks downward and pulls toward you and your left palm is pushed outward so they cross over (fig. 90). Your waist has turned to your right.

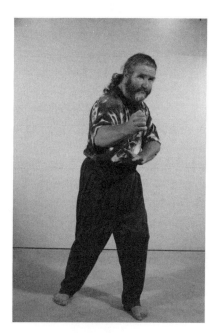

Figure 89

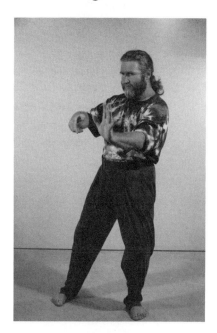

Figure 90

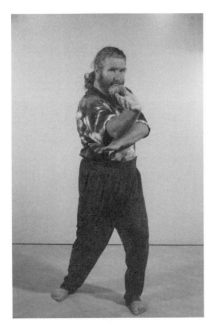

Figure 91

Stay weighted on the front foot as your waist turns to your left again and the right palm is thrust forward while the left palm is withdrawn to under your right elbow (fig. 91).

Turn your waist back to the right and pull your fight palm (hooked) back as your left palm cuts upward using the knife edge of the palm (fig. 92).

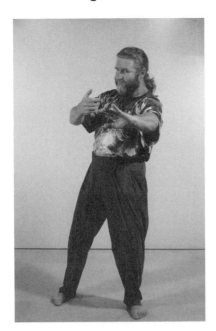

Figure 92

Turn your waist back to the left as your left palm pulls back and the right knife edge cuts upward (fig. 93). Take a step forward with your right foot so that you are now in the starting position for the reverse side (fig. 94).

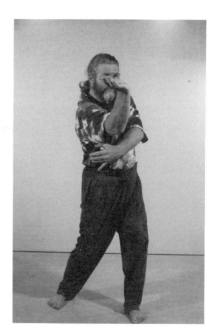

Figure 93

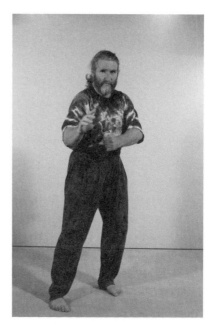

Figure 94

CHAPTER 8

SOLO KATA 8
Hammer Hand

The beginning posture is again the qigong for this kata. It is called the Hammer Hand because the palms and fist are not used in a fa-jing way; they simply hammer at arms and points, using the power of the waist to send them out centrifugally.

This qigong works upon the central nervous system. It has a great calming effect upon the whole system. When done slowly, it can be used to recuperate after illness or to calm you when you are agitated or angry.

HEALING

The kata works upon the liver, thus its use in combating anger. Its element is wood in Chinese medicine, and its time of day is between the hours of 1 A.M. and 3 A.M. The part of the body that it controls are the muscles and sinews.

THE QIGONG

With the right foot forward, stand with the weight

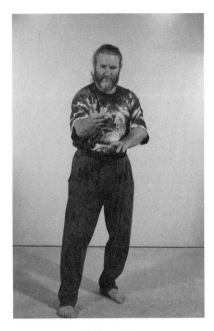

Figure 95

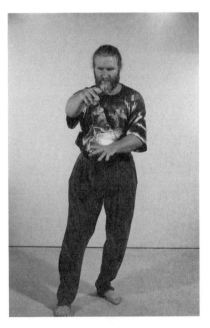

Figure 96

on the left foot and the hands held as in Figure 95. The left palm is facing downward while the right palm is facing upward. The breathing is all done through the nose with the tongue placed upon the hard palate. The eyes must look at (focus upon) the leading palm (in this case the right palm).

Inhale as you raise your right palm slightly upward and roll it over to palm down (fig. 96). Place your weight onto your right foot and turn your waist to your left as you again roll your right palm over to palm up and throw it downward to your left as you exhale. Your left palm will stay in the one position for the whole qigong (fig. 97). Turn your waist as far to your left as possible.

Inhaling and turning your waist to your right, sit back onto your rear leg and turn your right palm down and strike upward with it out to your right (fig. 98). This is one round.

You are now in the position to begin the inhalation again and the throwing down to your left. Do this 10 times on this side, then take a step forward and repeat the whole thing 10 times on the reverse side. Take a step forward again so that you are in the beginning position for the kata, with your right foot forward.

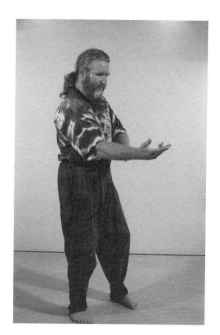

Figure 97

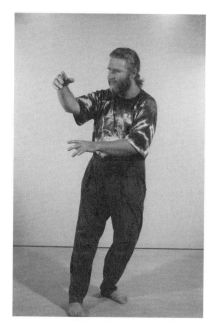

Figure 98

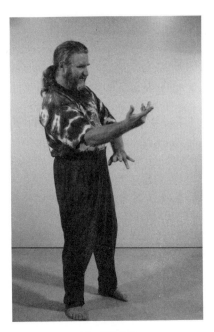

Figure 99

THE KATA

With right foot forward, turn the right hand to palm down. As you bring your weight forward and turn your waist to your left, the right palm again turns upward and strikes downward to your left. You are using the power of your waist in the same way that you did for the qigong, only now it is with much power and speed (fig. 99). Sit back onto your rear leg. Turning your waist to your right, thrust your right palm outward and up to your right, using the back of that palm. The left fingers are thrust forward as if jabbing into something (fig. 100).

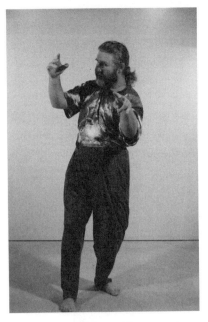

Figure 100

Turn your waist further to your right as your right palm begins to turn outward away from you to your right and curls over. Your weight has begun to come forward again (fig. 101). Bring your weight further forward and your right fingers downward as if digging something (fig. 102). Turn your waist to your left as you place the weight fully onto your right foot while your right fingers dig upward. The left palm is now under your right axilla (fig. 103). Pull the left palm outward as your waist turns further to your left. The right palm makes a hammer fist and is brought out as the waist turns (fig. 104). Sit back onto your rear foot as your waist turns violently to your right, thus thrusting centrifugally your right hammer fist to your right and down slightly (fig. 105). Take a step forward with your left

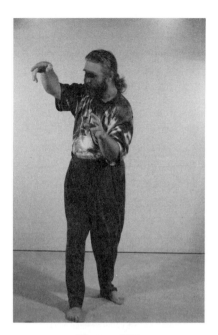

Figure 101

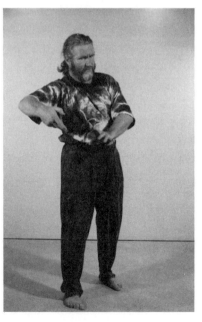

Figure 102

foot so that you are now in the position to do the whole kata on the reverse side.

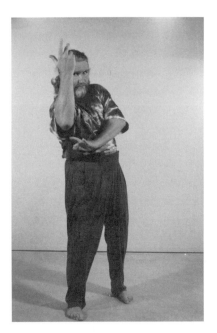

Figure 103

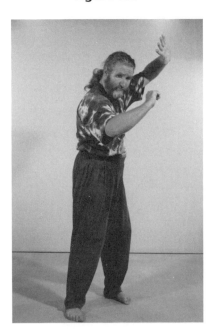

Figure 104

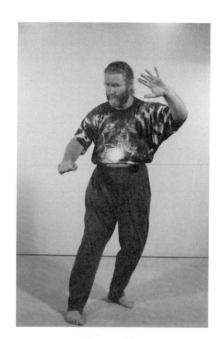

Figure 105

CHAPTER 9

SOLO KATA #9

Bumping Cutting Hand

The beginning posture is again the qigong for this kata, called Bumping Cutting Hand because of its less circular nature. It consists instead of a fa-jing bumping of the palms caused by the qi being used in a noncircular way.

This qigong is good for those who are affected by chronic fatigue syndrome, as it brings more yang energy to the body. It is not good for those who are already too yang, red-faced, get angry quickly, etc. It is more for those who are on the yin side.

I must add here that the qigong and the kata do different things. You may not wish to do the particular qigong associated with the kata for the above reasons, but that should not stop you from doing the actual kata.

HEALING

This kata works upon the lungs, and its time of day is between the hours of 3 A.M. and 5 A.M. Its Chinese medicine element is metal, and it controls the skin and body hair.

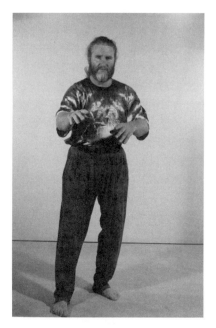

Figure 106

THE QIGONG

With the right foot forward and both hands facing downward at about chest height as in Figure 106, change your weight onto your right leg and thrust your fingers forward as you inhale (fig. 107). Continue to inhale as both your palms become yin shaped (relaxed), as in Figure 108. Breathe out as you lower your body and flex both palms downward (fig. 109). Your left palm is pushed over to your right as you inhale again and your right palm crosses over the top of the left (fig. 110). Sit back onto your rear leg as your right palm is thrust forward and your left is withdrawn upon the exhalation (fig. 111).

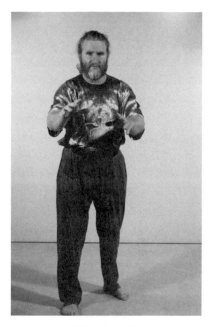

Figure 107

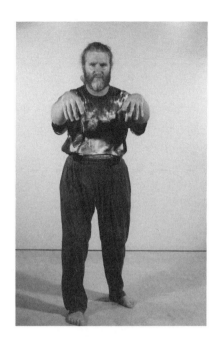

Figure 108

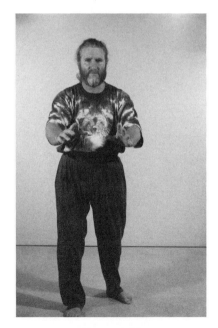

Figure 109

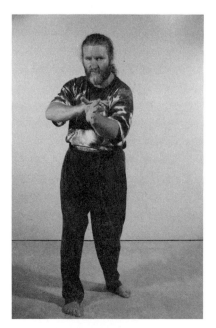

As the last bit of air is being exhaled, both your palms return to the beginning posture, ready to do it again. Do this 10 times and then take a step forward, ready to do it on the reverse side. Then take another step forward so that you are ready to begin the kata with the right foot forward.

Figure 110

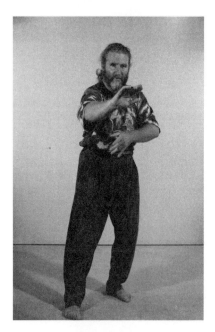

Figure 111

THE KATA

With the beginning posture the same as that of the qigong for this kata, step forward with your right foot and thrust both palms forward with a shake of the waist from left to right (fig. 112). The rear foot is dragged forward also so that the initial width of the stance is retained.

Thrust the backs of both wrists upward, also with a shake of the waist (fig. 113). With another fa-jing shake of the waist from left to right, thrust both palms downward as they flex (fig. 114).

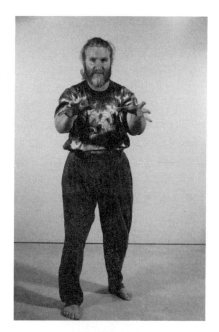

Figure 112

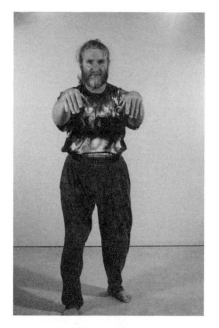

Figure 113

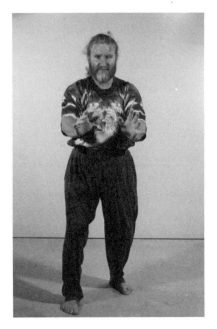

Figure 114

Push the left palm over to your right as the right palm is crossing over the top of it. Your waist has turned to your right (fig. 115). Sit back onto your rear leg as your right palm digs downward (fig. 116). Sit back fully as your waist turns to your left and your right palm leads upward in your center. Your left palm has risen, ready to strike (fig. 117). Turn your waist to your right and cut downward with the knife edge of your left palm (fig. 118).

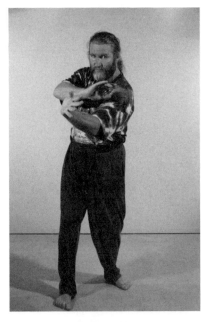

Figure 115

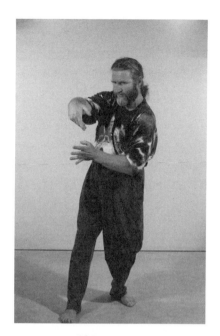

Figure 116

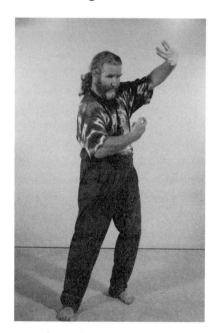

Figure 117

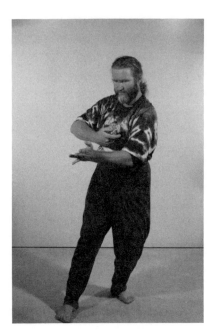

Take a step forward with your left foot so you are ready to begin on the reverse side.

Figure 118

DIM-MAK'S 12 MOST DEADLY KATAS

CHAPTER 10

SOLO KATA #10

Small Circle Hand

Once again, the beginning posture of this kata is also the qigong for this kata. This qigong will align the three centers or tantiens (psychic centers). In doing this, the whole organism will be in total harmony physically, mentally, and spiritually. In the self-defense area, it will enable the whole unit to act as one without thinking, as an animal does when attacked—with no logical thought.

The three centers are the upper center, just between the eyes on the forehead, the middle center at the solar plexus, and the lower center, about 3 inches below the navel on the midline.

HEALING

The Chinese medicine element for this kata is metal. It affects the large intestine while controlling the skin and body hair. The time of day for this kata is between the hours of 5 A.M. and 7 A.M.

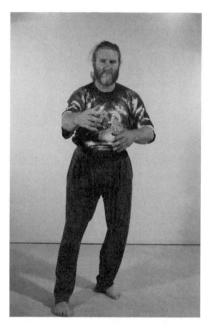

Figure 119

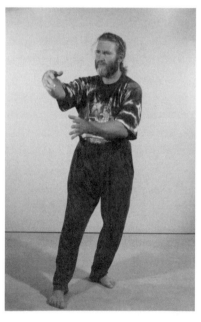

Figure 120

THE QIGONG

This qigong is one of the more simple, but that does not make it less effective. In fact this one is one of the more effective where inner stillness is concerned. By aligning the three centers, it brings the body, mind, and spirit into alignment, and therefore the whole organism is in a state of calm.

Stand with the right foot forward and the hands held in a sort of on-guard position (fig. 119). As the waist turns to your right, the right palm is relaxed, yin-shaped, while the left is flexed, or yang. You inhale on this movement as both palms are moved over to your right by the action of your waist (fig. 120). As you exhale, turn your waist to the left and bring both palms over to your left, with both changing state as they do this, i.e., the right becoming flexed while the left becomes relaxed (fig. 121). You repeat this process, turning the waist back to the right and changing the state of both palms while breathing in. You do this 10 times. Then step forward with your left foot and repeat the whole thing on the reverse side. Take another step with your right foot so that you are back with the right foot forward to begin the kata.

THE KATA

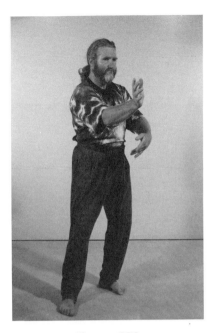

Figure 121

This kata begins exactly the same way the very first kata did. The only difference is in what the left hand is doing. As you move your weight to your right and turn your waist to your left, your right fist is thrust out and to your left. The left palm is now crossing over the top of the right wrist (fig. 122). Your weight has shifted onto your front leg. As you turn your waist to your right, your left palm

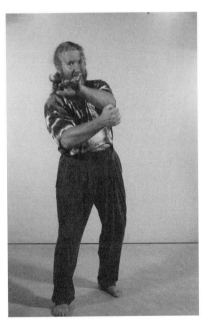

Figure 122

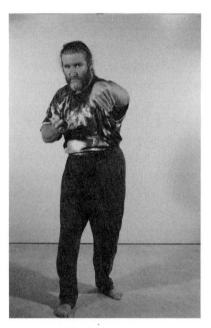

Figure 123

hooks over, ready to grab something, while your right tiger paw fist is withdrawn, ready to attack (fig. 123).

Your waist turns back to the left while your left palm pulls inward and your right fist attacks out to your left under your left palm (fig. 124).

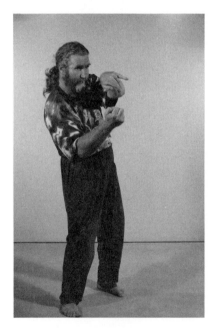

Figure 124

Your waist begins to turn back to the right as your left palm circles to attack to the right with its knife edge and the right palm crosses underneath the left wrist (fig. 125). Your weight has shifted back to the rear leg.

Your right palm hooks out to your right as your left palm circles up to your left, ready to strike downward (fig. 126). You are now weighted on your rear leg, which makes it easy to pick up your right knee as your right palm pulls down past it, followed by your left palm, which slams downward, as in Figure 127.

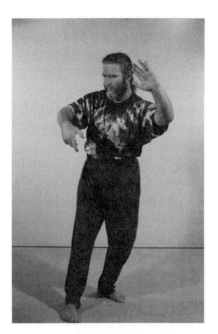

Figure 125

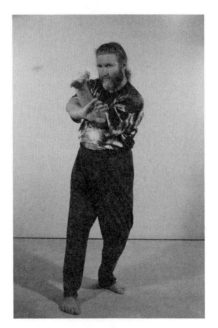

Figure 126

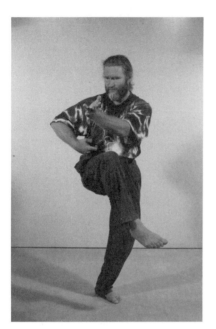

You place your right foot down and take a step forward with your left foot to repeat the whole kata on the reverse side.

Figure 127

CHAPTER 11

SOLO KATA #11

Eagle Shape Hand

The beginning posture of this kata is also the specific qigong for this kata. This qigong is used to build up the *wei qi*, or the qi that circulates over the surface of the body to protect it from disease and external attack.

HEALING

This kata is associated with the stomach, and it controls he flesh. The optimal time for this kata is between 7 A.M. and 9 A.M. Its TCM element is earth.

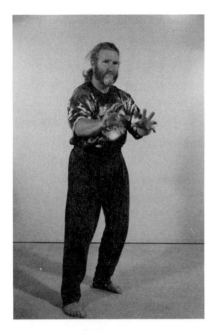

Figure 128

THE QIGONG

Stand with the right foot forward. The palms are held in the typical "eagle claw" way (fig. 128). The fingers are lightly stretched. The right palm is forward of the left palm, and the weight is placed onto the rear foot.

As you begin to inhale through your nose, the right palm turns upward and the waist turns slightly to your left (fig. 129). The waist now does a turn to your right, and the right palm turns to face downward (fig. 130).

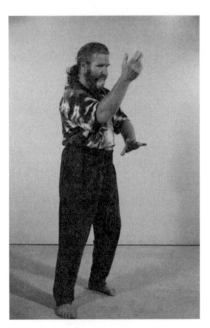

Figure 129

Raise the right palm as you continue to breathe in, and turn the waist fully to your right (fig. 131). Your waist turns to your left as you exhale, and your right palm turns to face upward as it moves down and to your left, gaining its power from the turning of the waist (fig. 132). Still on the exhalation, the waist turns to your right as your right palm moves in a circle upward and to your right as it turns to palm down.

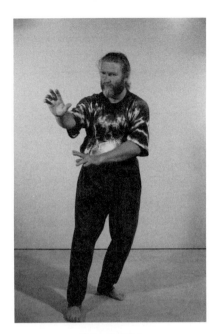

Figure 130

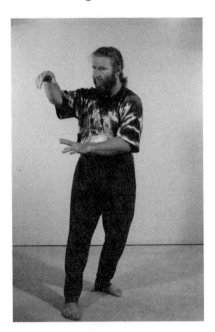

Figure 131

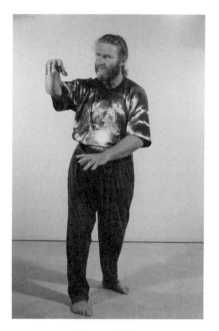

The turning of the palm from up to down and down to up is done slowly. It is not a sudden movement (fig. 133).

Figure 132

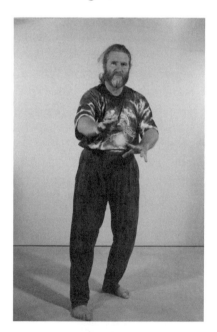

Figure 133

As the waist turns back to the left, no further than center, the right palm turns to palm down and claws downward upon the last bit of breath being exhaled (fig. 134). You do this 10 times, then reverse the stance and do it 10 times on the reverse side. Then take another step to bring your right foot forward so that you can begin the kata.

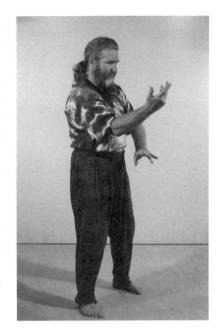

Figure 134

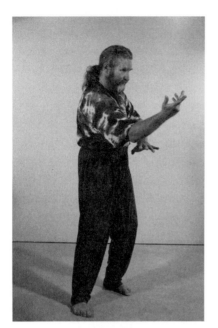

Figure 135

THE KATA

In the same beginning stance as for the qigong, turn your right palm up and strike downward to your left as your waist turns to the left. The weight remains on the rear foot (fig. 135). There is a compression on the right side of your abdomen (EX fig. 136).

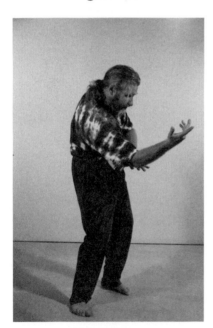

Figure 136

Your waist turns to the center (to the right of where it was), and the right palm circles counterclockwise to palm down and lifts upward (fig. 137). As the waist turns back to the left and the abdomen compresses, the right palm claws downward (fig. 138 and EX fig. 139).

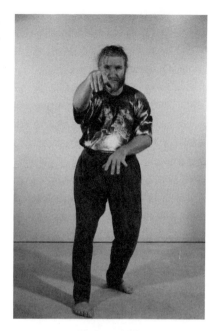

Figure 137

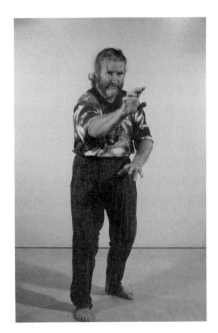

Figure 138

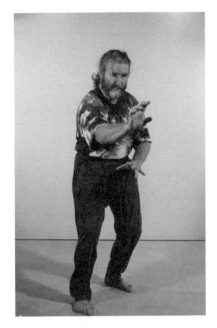

Figure 139

The waist turns further to your left, and the right palm continues the downward movement to your left (fig. 140). Your waist turns to your right as you transfer the weight onto your front leg and bring your left elbow up and to your right to strike. The right palm ends up under your left elbow (fig. 141). You now take a step forward with your left foot and perform the whole kata on the reverse side. This kata takes all of one-quarter of a second to perform. You breathe in just before you begin the first right palm movement and do the whole thing on the exhalation. (This is true for all of the 12 katas. The qigongs for each have their specific breathing techniques, but the katas are always done on the exhalation because the whole thing is a fa-jing movement.)

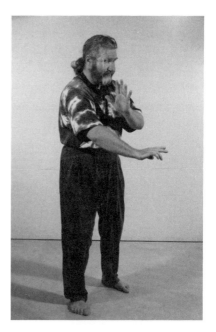

Figure 140

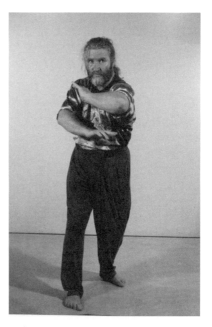

Figure 141

CHAPTER 12

SOLO KATA #12
Double Changing Hand

The beginning posture is also the specific qigong for this kata.

This qigong is used to balance the amount of yin and yang energy in the body. My view is that after having performed 11 quite explosive katas, we need something to rebalance the body so it returns to normal.

HEALING

This kata works upon the spleen and controls the flesh, and its time of day is between the hours of 9 A.M. and 11 A.M. So we have come full circle, having begun with the heart at 11 A.M. to 1 P.M. This kata's CTM element is earth.

THE QIGONG

This qigong is performed while breathing in through the nose and out through the mouth. The tongue is on the upper palate for the inhalation and on the lower palate for the exhalation.

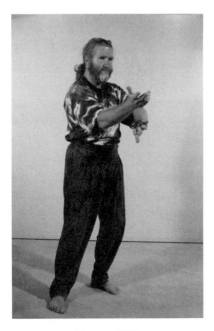

Figure 142

Stand with the right foot forward, weighted on the rear leg. Inhale as you turn your waist to the left. The right palm turns upward, while the left palm turns so that it is facing to your left. Bring some weight forward as both palms move over to your left (fig. 142). Sit back onto your rear leg as you turn your waist to your right and exhale. Your right palm turns to face down, while the left palm turns so that it is facing to the right. Both palms move over to your right (fig. 143).

You repeat this round 10 times, then take a step forward with your left foot and repeat it all on the reverse side.

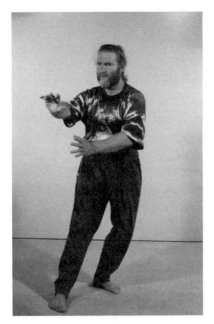

Figure 143

THE KATA

The first movement is exactly the same as the first movement of the first kata. The right fist attacks with tiger paw fist to your left as you shift your body to your right and turn your waist to your left (fig. 144). The weight has moved forward onto your front (right) leg. The right fist now turns so that the hammer part of the fist is facing to the right. The waist turns to your right, and at the same time your left palm attacks using the knife edge facing upward (fig. 145). Turning your waist to your left, you turn your right fist so that the hammer part is facing to your left, while turning the left palm so that it too is facing left. The power of the waist is used to take your palms over to your left (fig. 146).

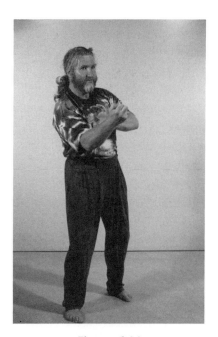

Figure 144

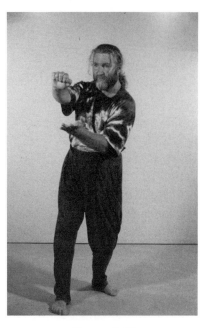

Figure 145

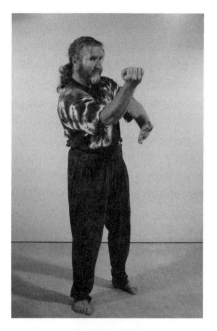

Figure 146

The waist turns back so that it is in the center line, while both palms now make tiger paw fists. Both tiger paw fists are thrust forward as you push your weight back onto the rear leg (fig. 147).

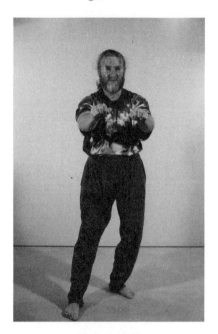

Figure 147

This next move is the only time in all of the katas where an inhalation is taken during the kata. You now open both palms and move them out to both sides (fig. 148). Hook both palms and move them together so that there are about 6 inches of space between the fingers of each palm (fig. 149). Still inhaling, you bring your weight forward onto the front foot and move the body to your left as you pull with both palms out to your right (fig. 150).

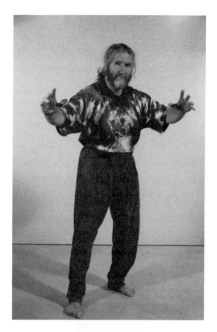

Figure 148

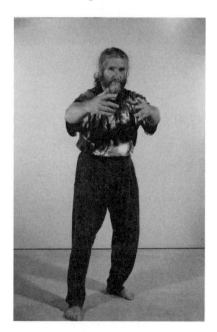

Figure 149

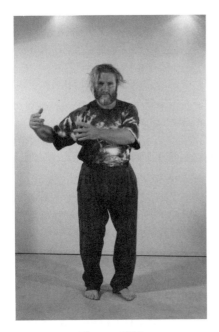

Figure 150

As you exhale through your mouth with the tongue on the lower palate, you turn your waist to your left and extend your elbow so that the inside of the elbow strikes forward (fig. 151). Now take a step forward with your left foot and do the whole kata on the reverse side.

• • •

This brings us to the end of the solo katas. They not only have a martial application, as you will see in the following chapter, but also a healing application through the qigongs and even the katas themselves.

These katas were invented and refined by men of genius, and who knows—some of them may have been women using men's names, as it was not kosher for women to invent martial arts back then. These people knew about the flows of qi

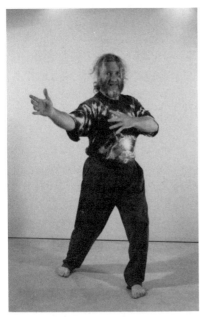

Figure 151

around the body, and all were Chinese doctors who knew about acupuncture. Every move we make causes an energy flow to happen within the body. Even a finger moving has to have qi to move, and that qi has to come from somewhere. It has to flow from the tantien to the portion of the body doing the work. The ancients worked out exactly what moves sent the qi to certain parts of the body, flowing through the 12 main acupuncture meridians in doing so, and thereby healing the associated organs. This is how taiji and bagwa work in the healing area, and so, too, do the 12 deadly katas of dim-mak work in the healing area. In the martial area, it is easier to see how the 12 katas work; the physical movement is greater than in the qigongs. The internal movement is still there but is now represented more physically.

Each of the previous 12 katas should take no more than two seconds to perform, and for the most part less than one second. They should be done as a fa-jing movement, and you must make some explosive noise with the mouth as you perform them.

Take it easy with these katas and try to understand them internally. Don't just learn the 12 in one day and think that you know them. These katas will work on your internal and external body and mind for your whole life, and you will learn everything that needs to be taught by just practicing them correctly.

Some time down the track, there will come a time when something changes inside, and you will then know the meaning of "the warrior within."

"How can you 'be' if you don't know?" This Chinese saying means that we cannot say that we are something when we do not truly know what it is that we are saying we are. Some people say that they are martial artists on the strength of learning a few katas and having a few dojo fights. Others learn some taiji kata or form in one year and then call themselves taiji experts. It takes *years* to "know" the martial arts. Once you have learned the physical movements, then you are only just beginning to open the door to see what is inside. When you have been practicing for at least five years, you can then say that you have entered the door and it has closed behind you. Then you look ahead and see the wealth of knowledge that the katas can teach you, and you realize that there is a lifetime's work there.

The above 12 katas will give you a lifetime's work, and you will learn much during that time. You will probably not know that you are learning much, as it will be mostly internal work that will spring upon you all of a sudden.

All of the katas make use of the hands only. There is an old saying in the internal martial arts: "Feet for standing, hands for fighting." And this is true. When you are young and robust physically, you are able to kick high and stand on one leg, but this only lasts for a short time. All of a sudden, you realize that you are no longer young. You then know that "youth" is only a brief time in your life, with the majority of your life spent being "old." We need a martial healing art that is not for young people, as we are only young for such a short time. The 12 deadly dim-mak katas make use of the palms only, with the feet serving to hold you up. These katas will hold you in good stead for the rest of your life, and as you progress, your healing skills will become greater, so that as you approach great old age, you will no longer need the martial arts skills, as they will have become one with the healing skills. And when our healing and martial become as one, then we become as one with God.

PART TWO

THE SAN-SAU OR KUMITE

*S*an-Sau, or *kumite* in Japanese, are two-person fighting sets of movements performed in order to learn what the kata means.

Many purists ask me why I mix the Japanese and the Chinese ways of speaking about the martial arts. They say that because I am teaching a Chinese-based martial art I should use the Chinese way of speaking.

I am not Chinese or Japanese and I will never be able to understand their cultures. There was a time when I thought that I could understand the Chinese way, and I wore Chinese clothes and tried to learn the Chinese language. Then I realized that I was only playing at being Chinese. I could never be Chinese, nor do I wish to be Chinese. I am happy with my own culture.

So nowadays I use the language that is most universal in describing what it is I am talking about. So if I use the word "dojo," for instance, everyone knows that I am talking about a training hall or space. If I use the word kata, martial artists know that I am talking about a series of movements depicting those of self-defense. Both of these words are Japanese, but one need not speak Japanese in order to understand them. I don't have to know the French language to know what an hors d'oeuvre is. Nor do I have to know German to know the meaning of kaputt.

I once had my photo on the front cover of an American martial arts magazine, and it caused much concern in the Chinese martial arts community in the United States, because they thought that it was not good to have someone who was not Chinese in such a prominent position. How could a non-Chinese, let alone someone from Australia, know something about the Chinese martial arts? Funny thing was, most of these Chinese martial artists were either born in the United States or had learned their martial arts there.

I take what I need from the Chinese or Japanese martial arts and use them; I don't have to become Oriental to know about their martial arts. The martial arts—Japanese, Chinese, Korean, Thai, Indian—have all become universal practices, with anyone—black, white, red, yellow, or green—having just as much chance of really knowing about them as the ethnic groups from whence the martial arts came.

The kumite that follow correspond to each of the 12 katas respectively, so all of the correct body movement has been learned already.

Please remember that when you begin working with a partner, there must never be any idea of competition. We in the martial arts should be above trying to be better than someone else, and that's all competition is. We learn these things for self-defense and the defense of our loved ones, not to show how good we are at the expense of another human being. Tournament fighting is just this and should never have been allowed to enter the realm of the martial arts. Push hands competitions (that silly area of little importance in one's taiji training when we use certain techniques to avoid being pushed or pulled over) are even worse. Those in the taiji area like to think that they are Taoists or follow some ancient, peaceful philosophy, and then they join in push hands competitions, the only outcome of which can be to show that they are better than someone else! How silly.

SAN-SAU #1

TRAINING THE HANDS

You have your partner hold two hard mitts (striking pads), as in Figure 152. You strike his right-hand mitt using the tiger paw fist with the knuckle of the longest finger protruding. The fist begins palm facing down, but as it strikes, it snaps upward and the one knuckle strikes the mitt, forcing it backward (figs. 153 and 154).

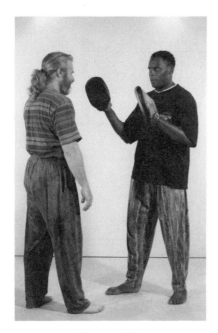

Figure 152

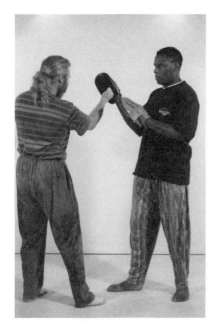

Figure 153

The one knuckle is withdrawn, making for a more normal fist shape. As the waist snaps back to your right, your right fist strikes the other mitt with the last three knuckles as the striking area (figs. 155 and 156).

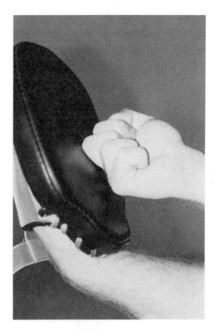

Figure 154

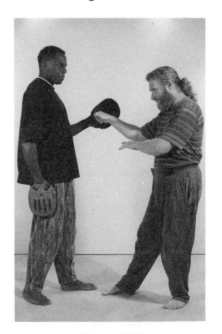

Figure 155

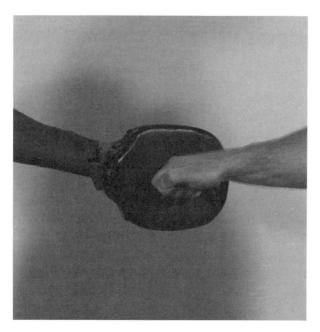

Figure 156

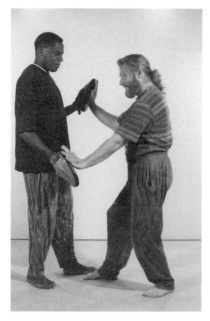

Figure 157

Your partner now moves his right-hand mitt to a lower position as you take a step inward with your right foot and strike both mitts with both of your open palms. The right palm strikes slightly before the left one. By the action of the elbows squeezing inward, the right palm is forced to do a clockwise circle as it strikes, and the left does a counterclockwise circle as it strikes (see figs. 157, 158, and 159).

Figure 157 shows the palms just before they strike, and Figure 158 shows the result of squeezing the elbows. Do this striking routine on both sides, i.e., now do it starting with the left fist.

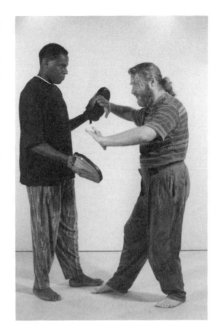

Figure 158

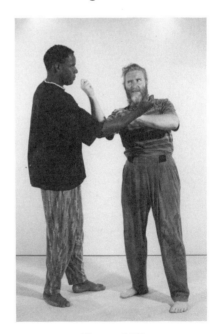

Figure 159

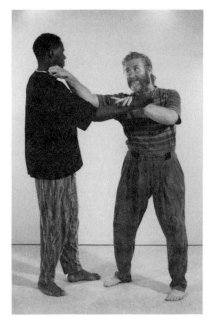

Figure 160

THE SAN-SAU (KUMITE)

This two-person set relates directly to Solo Kata No. 1 in Chapter 1.

You stand opposite your partner, who throws a straight right at your nose. You have your right foot forward. You change the weight to your right foot and turn your waist to your left, thus avoiding his strike. At the same time, as shown in Figure 160, your right tiger paw fist strikes to his Governor Vessel 26 (Gv 26) point (fig. 161). Your left hand is just near your right elbow guarding, ready to combat any reattack your opponent launches with his right hand.

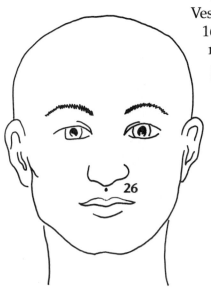

Figure 161

Your right fist now does a counterclockwise curve and, using the power of your waist turning to the right, strikes into his Stomach 9 (St 9) point (fig. 162). The left palm is there guarding his right hand. You now open your elbows and take a short step with your right foot to get in closer (fig. 163). As you squeeze your elbows, your right palm strikes to his Stomach 15 and 16 points on his left-hand side (fig. 164), while your left palm strikes to his Gall Bladder 24 (Gb 24) point on his right-hand side (fig. 165). The whole thing takes less than one second.

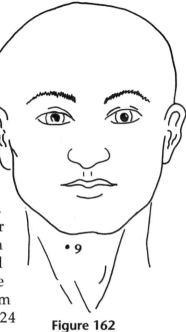

Figure 162

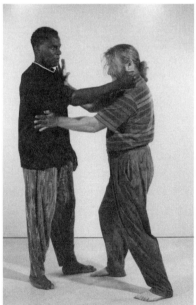

Figure 163

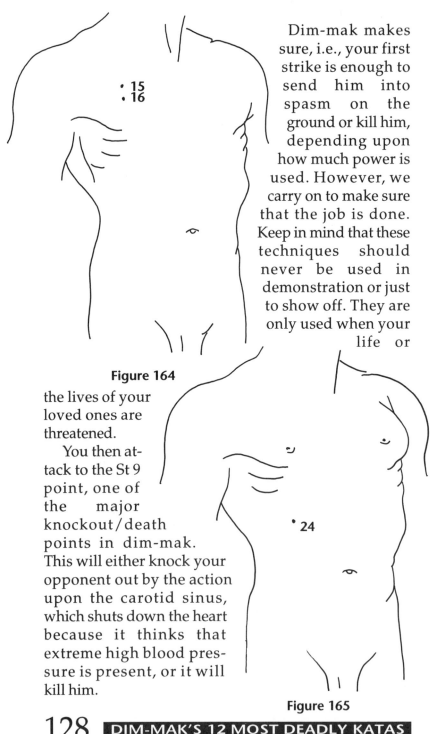

• 15
• 16

Dim-mak makes sure, i.e., your first strike is enough to send him into spasm on the ground or kill him, depending upon how much power is used. However, we carry on to make sure that the job is done. Keep in mind that these techniques should never be used in demonstration or just to show off. They are only used when your life or

Figure 164

the lives of your loved ones are threatened.

You then attack to the St 9 point, one of the major knockout/death points in dim-mak. This will either knock your opponent out by the action upon the carotid sinus, which shuts down the heart because it thinks that extreme high blood pressure is present, or it will kill him.

• 24

Figure 165

The strikes to the stomach points alone will cause the heart to stop, but when combined with Gb 24 they are devastating, as we have combined two heart stoppers. The St 15 and 16 points cause the heart to stop by physically affecting it directly, while Gb 24 affects the carotid sinus, which causes the cardioinhibitory center in the brain to tell the heart to stop.

As your partner throws a straight left punch to your nose (he has taken a step backward as he does this), you take a step forward, and as you do this, again avoid his strike and attack to his Gv 26 point with your left tiger paw fist. Now do the whole set on the reverse side. Having done this, you can then proceed to walk up and down the dojo doing the set. When you get to the end of the training hall, your partner becomes the person doing the techniques, and you become the attacker.

SAN-SAU #2

TRAINING THE HANDS

Your partner again has two hard mitts, one on each hand. His right-hand mitt is held at about face height, while the other is held at abdomen height (fig. 166).

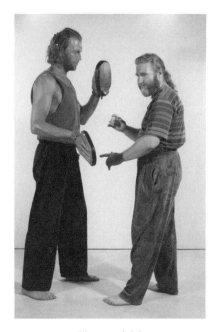

Figure 166

With your left foot forward, you move in and strike the upper mitt with your fingers just before your right palm strikes at the lower mitt. The time delay between strikes is only able to be "known" by you, as they strike almost simultaneously. But beware—work your fingers up slowly, as they can be damaged if this strike is done incorrectly. Allow the fingers to make contact with the mitt, not straightened but as a claw, so that there is some give if you should make contact with a hard bony area (fig. 167).

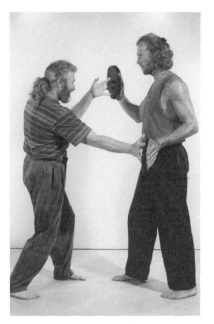

Figure 167

Your partner now turns his right-hand mitt so that the striking area is facing to his left. You now allow the power from the first strike to rebound into the next strike, which is a penetration punch gaining its power from the waist (fig. 168).

Your partner now brings his left-handed mitt into play, turning it toward you. You do a change step, i.e., bring your left foot back and then take your right foot forward. As soon as your right foot is placed forward, your right palm does a backfist strike to the mitt, again gaining its power from the waist (fig. 169). Remember, it is the pulling back of the wrist that causes the fist to have whipping power and not necessarily the thrust forward.

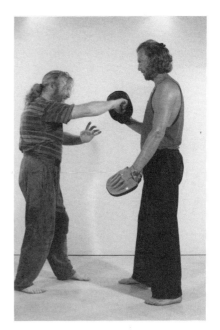

Figure 168

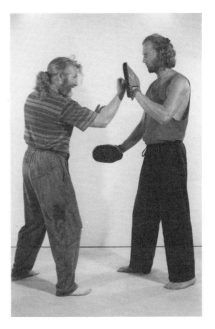

Figure 169

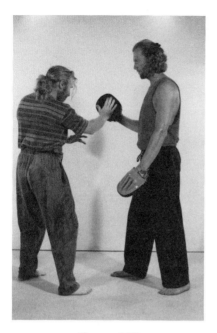

Figure 170

Again, using the fajing power of the waist, you strike the right-handed mitt, which has been turned appropriately, using your left palm (fig. 170).

THE SAN-SAU (KUMITE)

This two-person set relates directly to the Solo Kata No. 2 in Chapter 2.

Stand opposite your partner with your left foot forward. He throws a right straight at your face. You barge in with your left foot forward as your left fingers poke toward his carotid sinus or Stomach 9 point, at the right side of his neck. This has the effect of blocking his attack and causing a knockout by the affect of St 9 upon the carotid sinus, which in turn causes the heart to slow down or stop. It does not matter if your left palm goes on the outside of his arm or the inside, you still block his attack and attack to

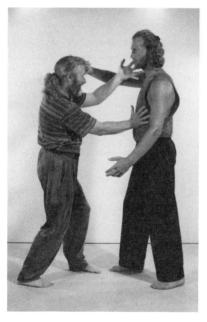

Figure 171

the neck. A split second later, your right palm, attacks to the Gb 24 point on the left side of his abdomen (fig. 171).

Your waist now shakes violently, causing your right penetration punch to attack to his left temple or Gall Bladder 3 (Gb 3) point. All of the gall bladder points are knockout points that affect the carotid sinus and the cardioinhibitory center in the brain, which causes the heart to either stop or slow down. As you do this, your left palm, also taking its power from the movement of the waist, strikes his right forearm outward. This strike happens a fraction of a second before the temple strike and is regarded as a "set-up" point strike, causing his energy or qi to be drawn to the area of the inner wrist (fig. 172).

You again shake your waist. As you do this, your left foot is withdrawn, and your palm again strikes the inner side of his wrist, causing

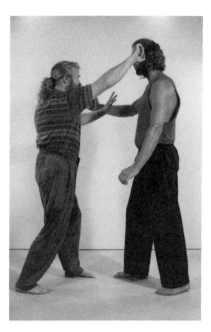

Figure 172

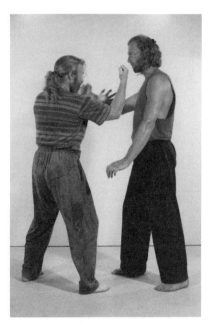

Figure 173

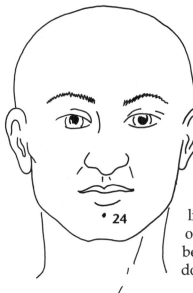

Figure 174

an energy drainage. As your right foot comes forward. (this has all taken a split second), you strike his Conceptor Vessel (Cv 24) point with your right backfist (fig. 173). Cv 24 is situated in the center-line of the body just over the chin in the indentation between the chin and lower lip (fig. 174). This has the effect of causing his qi or energy to be totally scattered, so that he does not know where he is.

You finish off with a right palm slap to his neurological shutdown point No. 3 at the back of the neck, thus the waist again shakes violently and again the left palm strikes the inside of his right wrist. Your right palm is placed so that the longest finger lies just under his chin bone. This will cause the nervous system to shut down, a phenomenon that occurs only in hum-ans (fig. 175). You now have your right foot for-ward, ready to do the whole thing on the reverse side, with your partner attacking with a left straight to your face.

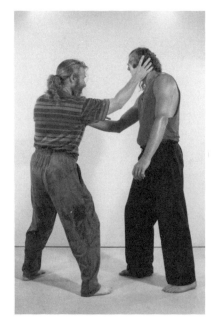

Figure 175

CHAPTER 15

SAN-SAU #3

TRAINING THE HANDS

In this set, we only make use of the palms and not the fist. Your partner holds one hard mitt facing toward you at about face height. You have your right foot forward as you step in and strike the mitt using the dim-mak claw (described in detail in my earlier book, *Advanced Dim-Mak: the Finer Points of Death-Point Striking)*. The palm is concave so that the fingers make contact first. It is the fingers that are doing the damage here (fig. 176).

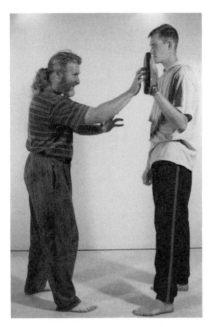

You turn your waist to your left and then turn back to the right as your right palm turns facing toward you and you strike with the back of it, taking the power from the turning of the waist (fig. 177).

Figure 176

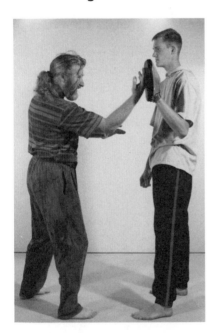

Figure 177

Again, you turn your waist to your left so that you are able to use a fajing movement to the right, which thrusts your right fingers inward. Be careful here not to hurt your fingers. Build this one up slowly (fig. 178).

Bring your right foot back and as your left foot comes forward, strike the mitt with your left palm (fig. 179).

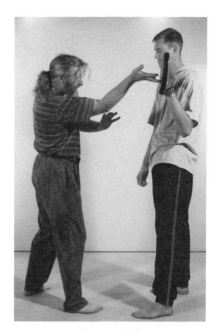

Figure 178

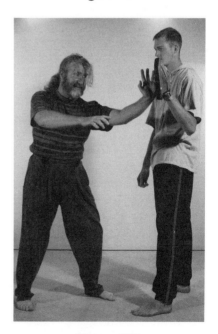

Figure 179

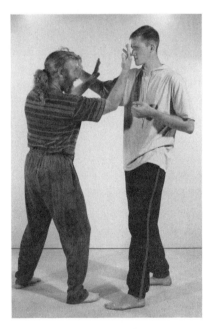

Figure 180

Figure 181

THE SAN-SAU (KUMITE)

This two-person set relates directly to the solo set in Chapter 3. Your partner attacks you with a right straight or hook. (It really doesn't matter what type of attack he uses, as you have to be able to defend against all attacks.) The left palm will take care of this attack as you step in with your right foot and claw to his eyes with your right fingers (fig. 180).

Using the built-up power and fa-jing generated by your waist, you now shake your waist violently, causing your right palm to be cracked onto the right side of his face. Your right first knuckle is placed over his cheekbone while the knuckles of your fingers are placed over his right eyebrow (fig. 181). This will cause a neurological shutdown. (This strike is, in fact, neurological shutdown No. 1).

Again using the shaking of your waist,

your right fingers now spear into the pit of his neck to the point called Conceptor Vessel 22 (Cv 22). This in itself is a death-point strike (fig. 182).

Now you take hold of his left forearm at the wrist and hammer the wrist toward you, causing an energy drainage by the action upon the points Heart 5 (H 5) and Lung 8 (Lu 8). You have also changed step, bringing your right foot back and then taking your left foot forward. Your left palm slams into his neck at St 9. This causes the heart to stop by the action of the carotid sinus and vagus nerve, which control the heart rate (fig. 183).

You end up with your left foot forward, ready to begin on the reverse side with your partner throwing a left-handed attack to your face.

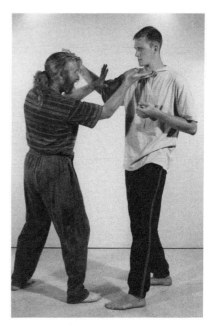

Figure 182

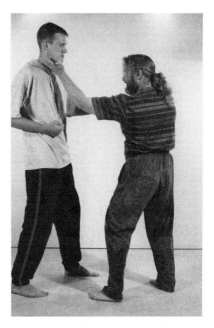

Figure 183

CHAPTER 16

SAN-SAU #4

TRAINING THE HANDS

This is one of the shorter kumite; however, it is also one of the most deadly, so be careful in your training.

The only training that this kumite involves is to slam the heel of your palm into the mitt using the power of your waist in a centrifugal motion. This is not done in a fa-jing way, but rather, the waist turns and the hands follow through and do not snap back as for fa-jing. The arms must be held extremely relaxed so that the maximum power is in the hands. So be careful with this one, as the power that is generated is tremendous and people have been hurt in training by not realizing how much power can be obtained simply by relaxing the arms and turning the waist.

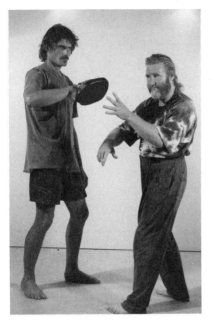

Have your partner hold the mitt facing slightly upward. You raise your palm as in Figure 184. Now, by the turning of your waist from the center, your arm is thrown onto the mitt with great force (fig. 185). Even with the mitt on his hand, when this strike is done correctly it will be too much power for your partner. The energy goes right through the mitt and damages his hand, so pull it.

Figure 184

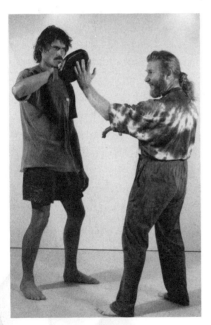

Figure 185

144

THE SAN-SAU (KUMITE)

This two-person set relates directly to Solo Kata No. 4 in Chapter 4. You stand with your left foot forward. Your partner throws a low right hook to your lower left rib area. You step to your right with your left foot and slam just above the inside of his right elbow joint with your right palm. This is dangerous, as it can cause extreme nervous damage to the whole body, let alone taking out his arm! Look at the left palm—it is sneaking up over the top of the right palm (fig. 186).

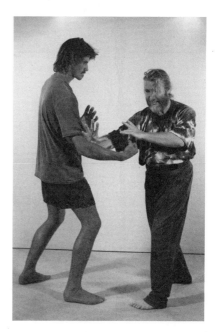

Figure 186

Your left palm now strikes to his Stomach 9 point at the right side of his neck (fig. 187). This causes his heart to either stop, falter, or slow down dramatically, resulting in a knockout. Your left palm continues to wrap around his neck (fig.188). You pull his head downward as your right palm rises high (fig. 189).

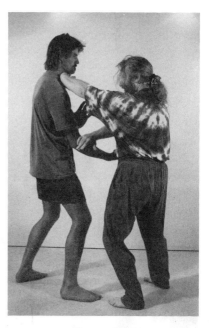

Figure 187

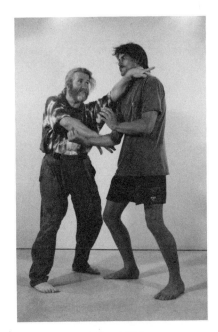

Figure 188

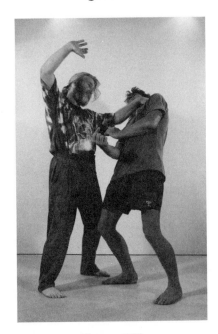

Figure 189

Finish by cutting down across his thyroid cartilage (Adam's apple), which, if you did it for real, would kill him instantly (fig. 190).

You take a step forward with your right foot and out to your right as he attacks this time with his low left hook and you do the whole kumite on the reverse side.

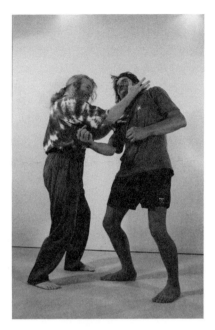

Figure 190

SAN-SAU 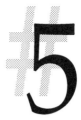 5

TRAINING THE HANDS

This set uses multiple point strikes as well as "set-up" point strikes. Set-up points are those that are not necessarily the final strike, but those that help to make the major point strikes more effective. We could for instance, drain qi from the heart and lungs before the major strike. This causes the attacker's body to have no resistance to the major point strike, as his seat of power has been drained of energy.

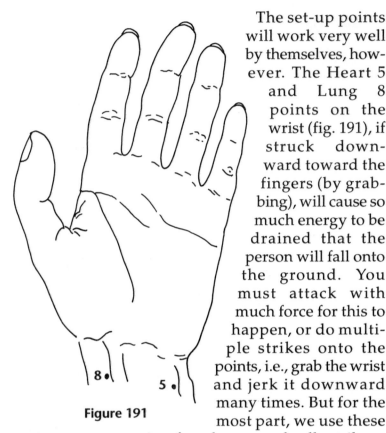

The set-up points will work very well by themselves, however. The Heart 5 and Lung 8 points on the wrist (fig. 191), if struck downward toward the fingers (by grabbing), will cause so much energy to be drained that the person will fall onto the ground. You must attack with much force for this to happen, or do multiple strikes onto the points, i.e., grab the wrist and jerk it downward many times. But for the most part, we use these points as set-up points for other, more deadly strikes.

Figure 191

Your partner holds two mitts. You stand with right foot forward and strike his left-handed mitt with your right snake fingers (fig. 192). Be careful here, as you might damage your fingers doing it incorrectly. Be sure that when you make contact, the fingers are not held rigid or extended as in Figure 193. They must make contact (fig. 194) so that if you hit something hard, there will be some "give." The strike is done as usual with a fa-jing shake of the waist to cause the fingers to be whipped outward; you should not just extend your arm.

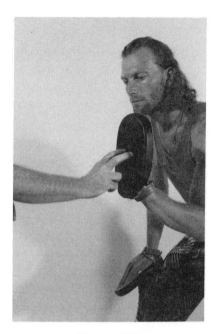

Figure 192

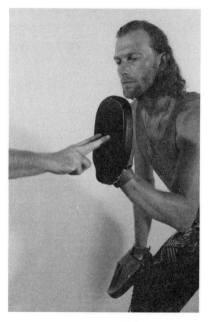

Figure 193

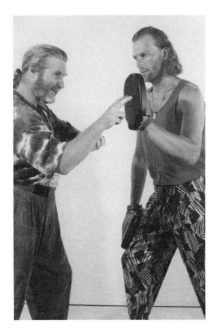

Using the power from the rebound of that last fa-jing shake, you again attack his left mitt with your right tiger paw fist, facing upward (fig. 195).

Figure 194

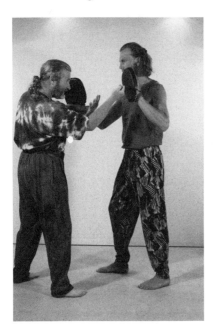

Figure 195

Take a left step to the front and out to your left and strike his right mitt with a downward palm strike. This is not a fa-jing strike, but rather a power strike using the waist with the palm following (fig. 196).

Your left palm now strikes to the left mitt using the knife edge (fig. 197).

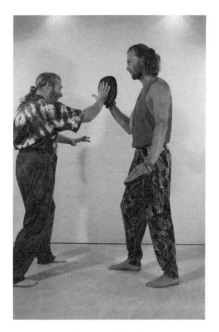

Figure 196

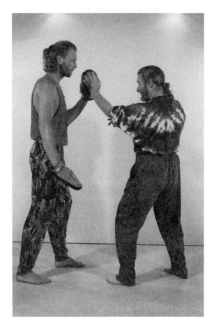

Figure 197

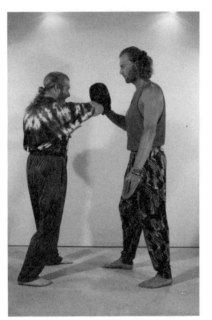

Using the power of your waist, you strike his right mitt with your right elbow. Keep your palm facing downward, as this will ensure that you are striking with the correct part of your elbow (fig. 198).

Figure 198

THE SAN-SAU
(KUMITE)

This two-person set relates directly to Solo Kata No. 5 in Chapter 5.

You stand with your right foot forward as your partner throws a right straight at your face. This first technique comes from the taijiquan movement of sit back ready (fig. 199). Your left palm will explode outward to block and attack his oncoming forearm, sliding up the inside of his forearm, thus setting up the next strike. A split second later, your right fingers attack to his eyes using the power of your waist (fig. 200). Notice that you have moved your weight to your right to also avoid his attack.

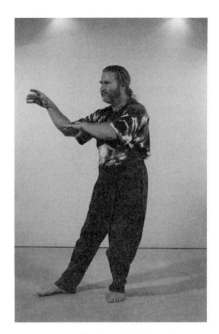

Figure 199

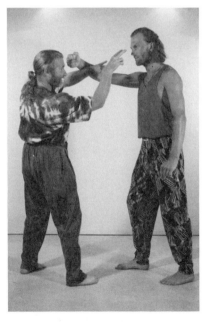

Figure 200

Figure 201

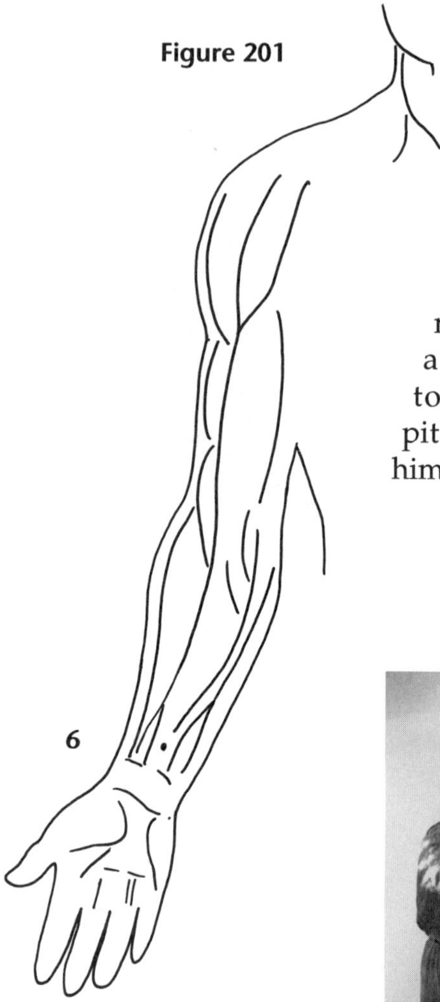

Rebounding off that last attack, you again shake your waist and again attack the set-up point on the inside of his forearm called Neigwan or Pericardium 6. (fig. 201). Your right fist turns over into a tiger paw fist to attack to the Cv 22 point in the pit of his neck. This will kill him (fig. 202).

6

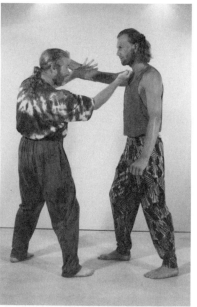

Figure 202

Take a step to your left diagonally as you strike the outside of your opponent's left forearm over to your right as you slap downward onto Gall Bladder 14 (Gb 14), just above the center of his eyebrow by 1 inch. This must be a downward strike to cause his heart to slow or stop. Your left palm struck the outside of his right forearm, sliding upward on the forearm to set up this Gb 14 strike (fig. 203).

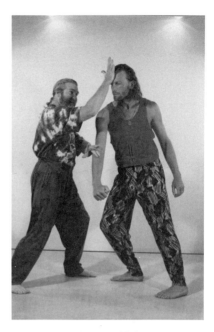

Figure 203

Grab his right arm (your partner might like to strike at you with his right arm to make it easier to grab) with your right palm and strike to his "mind point" (an "extra" acupuncture point on the back of the jaw that, when struck in toward the backbone, will prevent the signals from the central nervous system from getting to the brain) on his right jaw. For the mind point to work as a knockout point, the strike must be back toward the backbone (fig. 204).

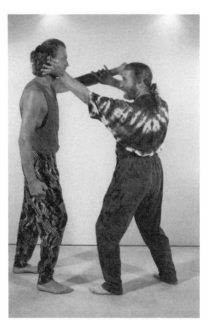

Figure 204

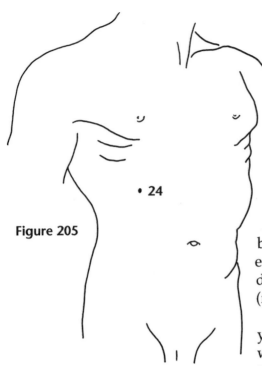

Figure 205

• 24

Using the power of your waist turning to your right, you bring your right elbow across to strike straight into his Gall Bladder 24 (Gb 24) point (fig. 205), about 2 inches below his nipple on either side. This is a death-point strike (fig. 206).

You now have your left foot forward, ready to do the whole thing on the reverse side.

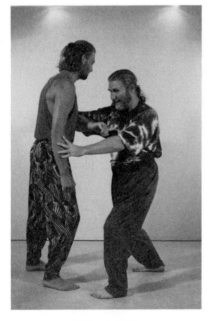

Figure 206

CHAPTER 18

SAN-SAU #6

TRAINING THE HANDS

Again, we use the snake fingers, as in the previous chapter. You strike at the mitt with your right fingers and with your right foot forward (fig. 207).

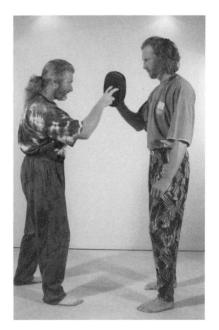

Turning your waist to your right, you strike the mitt with your left palm, using the knife edge (fig. 208).

Figure 207

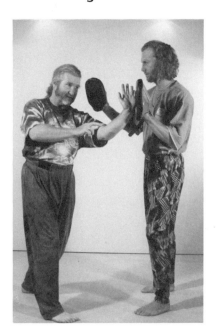

Figure 208

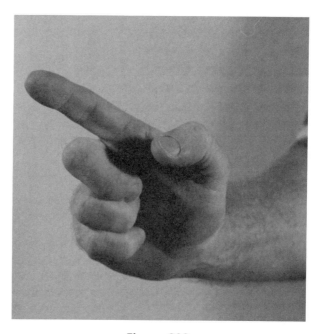

Figure 209

Your partner will have to turn the mitt to an angle for this next strike. The striking parts of your right palm are the thumb and forefinger. The hand is held as in Figure 209. Strike the mitt with a shake of your waist that causes the palm to be thrust out onto the mitt. Be careful with this one, as it could damage your fingers if done incorrectly (fig. 210).

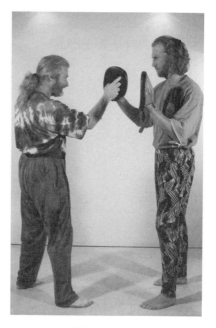

Figure 210

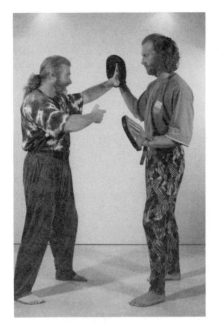

Figure 211

Do a change step, and with your left foot forward, strike the right-handed mitt with your left heel palm (fig. 211).

THE SAN-SAU (KUMITE)

This set is directly related to Solo Kata No. 6 in Chapter 6. Your partner attacks with a right straight to your face again. You have your right foot forward as you avoid his attack by changing your weight over to the right and blocking his attack with your left palm, which slides back up the inside of his forearm. This is the set-up strike. Your right fingers are poked into his eyes again, as in the previous chapter (fig. 212).

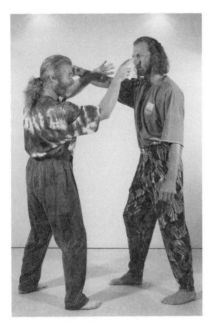

Figure 212

Your partner tries to attack you with his left fist to your face. You grab his left wrist with your right palm and jerk it violently, hammering upon Lung 8 and Heart 5 points to drain his power (qi). A split second later, your left palm attacks to his Small Intestine 16 (Si 16) point, located at the side of his neck in the centerline where the neck makes contact with the shoulder (figs. 213 and 214). Si 16 is a death-point strike and, at the very least, will cause the attacker to feel so ill that he cannot carry on with the attack. Combined with the qi drainage of H 5 and Lu 5, this is a devastating strike.

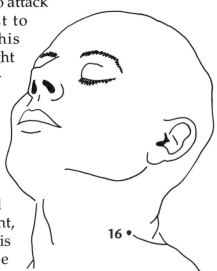

Figure 213

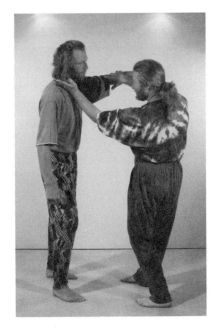

Figure 214

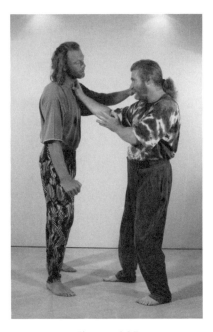

Figure 215

Now for the finale. With the fa-jing of your waist turning to your left, your right fingers strike to two points. With the hand held in the position described previously and shown in Figure 209, you thrust your thumb into the pit of his neck (Cv 22), while the index finger strikes into St 9. Both of these points are death points, but when they are used together, there is no possibility of resuscitation (fig. 215).

Your right palm grabs around the back of his neck as you do a change step. Your left palm strikes up into his forehead as your right palm pulls forward violently, thus breaking his neck (fig. 216). Be really careful when training with this one.

You are now in a position to begin this kumite on the reverse side with your left foot forward.

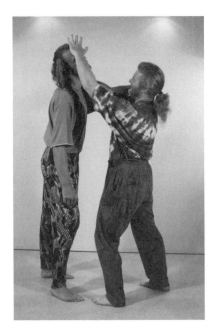

Figure 216

CHAPTER 19

SAN-SAU #7

TRAINING THE HANDS

Your partner holds the mitt facing to his right. You step to your left with your left foot and slam the mitt with your right backfist, using the power of the waist shaking from right to left (fig. 217).

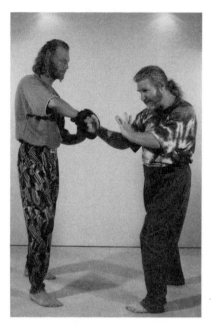

Your partner turns the mitt toward you as you strike it using the heel of your right palm, again using a fa-jing movement from your waist (fig. 218).

Figure 217

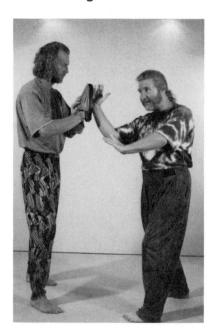

Figure 218

The mitt is held a little higher as you strike it using the heel of your left palm, facing downward (fig. 219).

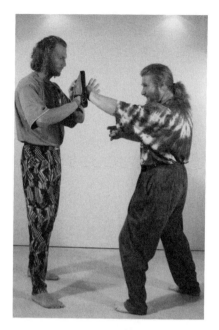

Figure 219

THE SAN-SAU (KUMITE)

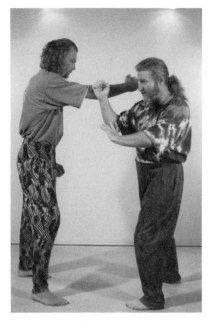

Figure 220

This set is directly related to Solo Kata No. 7 in Chapter 7. You are standing with your left foot forward. Your partner attacks with a right straight to your face. You step to your left with your left foot and attack to his right forearm with your right backfist, aiming at Colon 10 (Co 10), as in Figure 220. Figure 221 shows the exact location of the point, which will cause great sickness in the lower abdomen, causing your opponent to lose his will to carry on with the attack. If you strike to this point too many times, it will result in a knockout.

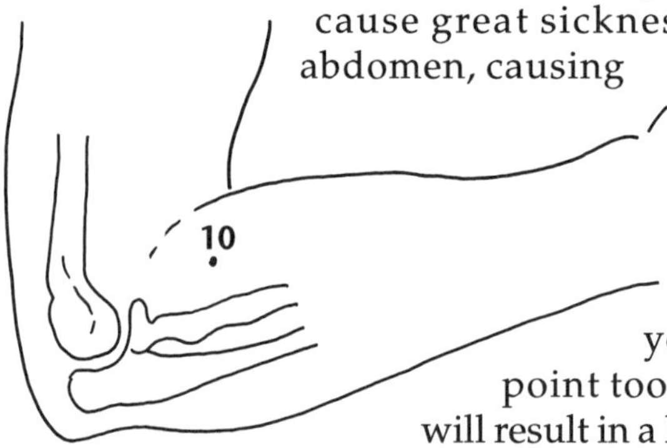

Figure 221

Your right palm grabs his right wrist as, with a shake of the waist, you use your left palm to strike his arm just above his elbow. This not only breaks the arm but attacks to Colon 12 (Co 12), just above the elbow on the outside of the arm, causing the same side of his body to become very weak (fig. 222).

Controlling his right arm with your left palm, you turn your waist to your left and strike him across his neck at Cv 22 (fig. 223).

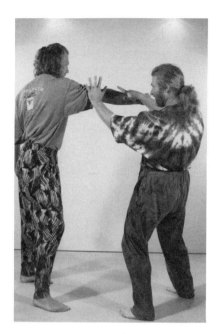

Figure 222

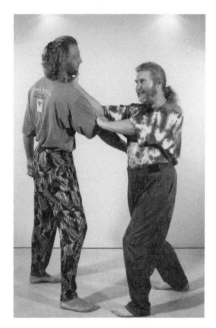

Figure 223

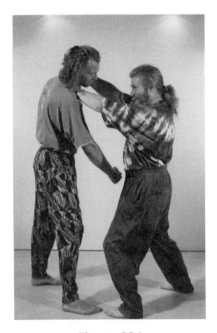

Figure 224

Your right palm grabs across the back of his neck, and as you pull him forward your left palm strikes again across Cv 22 (fig. 224). Cv 22 is a death point from which there is no return.

Your left palm now reverses and slams him in the back to pull him forward again. Your right palm now strikes up under his nose at Governor Vessel 26 (Gv 26), which, being a nerve attack, causes his whole body to go into spasm (fig. 225).

Your partner throws a left attack, so you step forward with your right foot and do the whole thing on the reverse side.

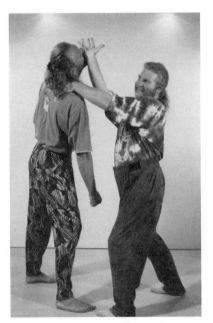

Figure 225

CHAPTER 20

SAN-SAU #8

TRAINING THE HANDS

Here we make use of the back of the palm to attack. There is one rule when doing this: do not strike with the middle of the back of the palm; turn it to either side so that a flat area is exposed. If you look at your palm, you will notice that it is not flat across the back but curved, with two flat sides. Turning the palm in either direction causes one of these flat areas to be exposed to the striking target, thus lessening the chance of damaging one of the small bones in the palm. Figures 226 and 227 show the correct way to strike with the back of the palm.

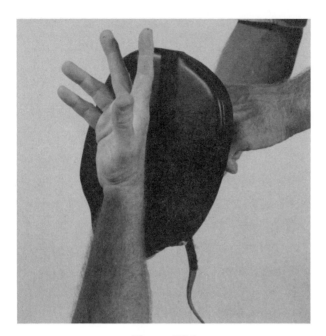

Figure 226

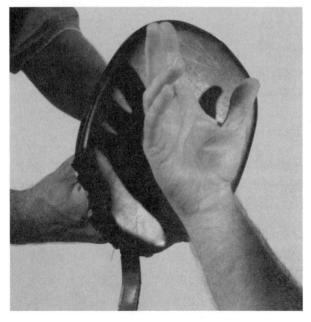

Figure 227

We also use the snake finger strike as in Chapter 17, so I will not cover that again. Your partner holds the mitt as shown, and you strike using the hammer part of your fist (fig. 228).

THE SAN-SAU (KUMITE)

This set is directly related to Solo Kata No. 8 in Chapter 8. Your partner throws a low right hook at your lower left rib area. You have your right foot forward as you slam the inside of his right elbow just above the joint with the back of your right palm. This is not a fa-jing shake but a move wherein palm follows the waist's movement to your left and takes its power from that (fig. 229).

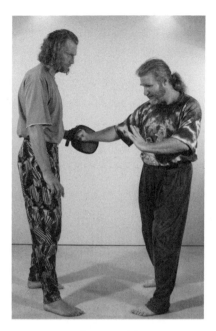

Figure 228

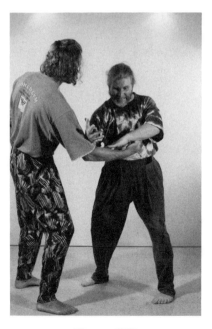

Figure 229

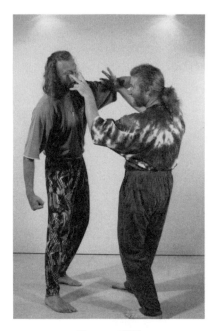

Figure 230

He now attacks with his left fist high. You turn your waist to your right, and your right palm again strikes to just above the inside of his left elbow. A split second after this, your left fingers strike to his eyes. The strike to the inside of his elbow is particularly nasty, as it causes his nervous system to go into spasm at the most and will take out his arm at the least (fig. 230).

You now move in by taking a right step in to close any gap between you and your opponent. Your right palm snakes over the top of his left arm (fig. 231) and then locks his shoulder and elbow (fig. 232). Be careful with this one, as a slight exaggeration of the movement could twist his shoulder off.

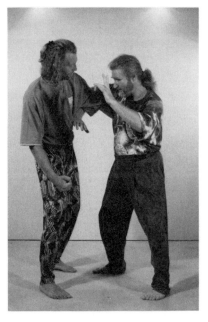

Figure 231

Your left palm grabs his left wrist and pulls it upward as your waist turns to your left and your right hammer fist is cocked, ready (fig. 233). Turning your waist to your right, as shown in Figure 234, you strike with your right hammer fist at Liver 13 (Liv 13). Figure 235 shows the exact location of Liver 13. A strike to this point attacks the liver, causing massive internal bleeding and liver damage, which means instant death.

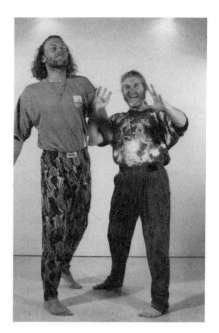

Figure 232

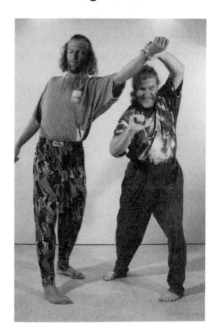

Figure 233

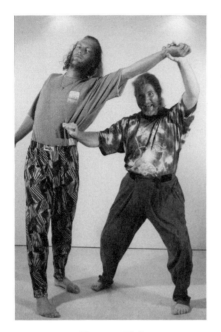

You now change your footing and repeat the whole set on the reverse side.

Figure 234

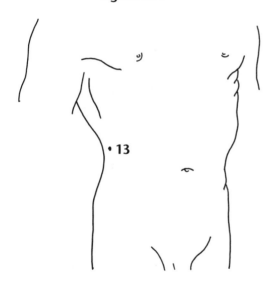

• 13

Figure 235

CHAPTER 21

SAN-SAU #9

TRAINING THE HANDS

You should be a little cautious with this first strike, as it makes use of the fingers. Make sure that when you strike with the tips of the fingers they are not held rigid but rather in the "claw" configuration. And when you make contact, be sure that there is some "give" in your fingers.

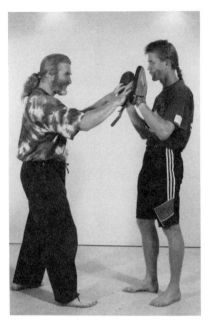

Figure 236

Your partner holds the two mitts toward you. You have your right foot forward as you step in and strike the mitt with both of your palms, using the fingers to strike (fig. 236).

Your partner points the mitts slightly downward as you strike upward with the backs of your palms. The power for this move comes from your waist (fig. 237).

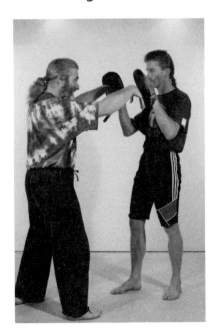

Figure 237

Now the mitts are both turned outward as you hammer down onto each mitt with both palms using the knife edges (fig. 238).

THE SAN-SAU (KUMITE)

This san-sau is directly related to Solo Kata No. 9 in Chapter 9. Your partner attacks with either hand to your face. You step in with your right foot and simultaneously block and attack with your fingers to the pit of his neck at Cv 22. His attack can either be on the closed side or the open side; it does not matter, as your barging in will enable you to block his attack (fig. 239). Note that this is not a simultaneous strike with both palms. The right palm makes contact slightly before the left one. This enables you to make use of the turning of your waist in a fa-jing movement.

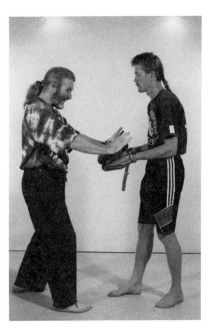

Figure 238

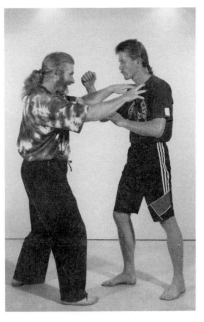

Figure 239

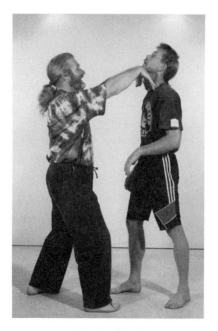

Figure 240

Again turning your waist to your left and then violently right, slam both palms (right one first) into the underside of his chin, thus forcing his head and neck to be forced backward violently (fig. 240).

Again with a left/right waist shake, slam both palms (right one first) downward into both of your opponent's Stomach 12 points (St 12) at the center of the collar bone on the inside. This will cause great qi drainage and take away his will to fight (fig. 241).

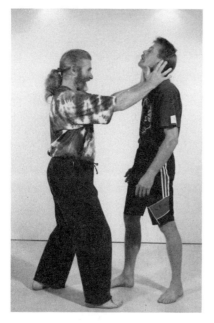

Figure 241

With a very explosive right/left shake of your waist, you first (on turning to the right) slap into the side of his neck at his right St 9 point, which causes knockout or death (fig. 242). On the other part of this shake (to your left), your right palm snakes upward around his neck (fig. 243). As shown in Figure 244, your right palm now snakes fully around his neck, thus turning it upward. Your left palm has also raised up. This will break his neck.

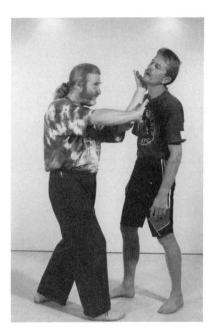

Figure 242

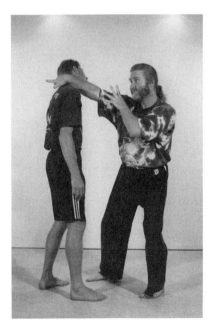

Figure 243

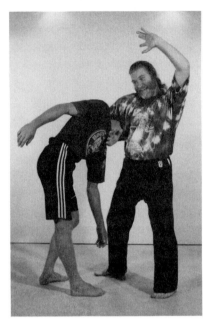

You finish by slamming across his Adam's apple (thyroid cartilage) with the knife edge of your left palm, thus causing instant death (fig. 245).

Your partner takes a step back and again attacks with either hand. Now take a left step in toward him and repeat the whole thing on the reverse side.

Figure 244

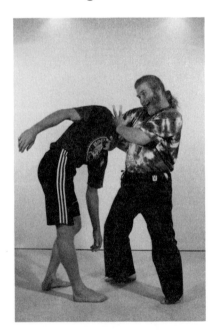

Figure 245

CHAPTER 22

SAN-SAU #10

TRAINING THE HANDS

Not so much training of the palms is necessary by this time, as we are up to the tenth set, and by now you have trained the palms, bar a few techniques.

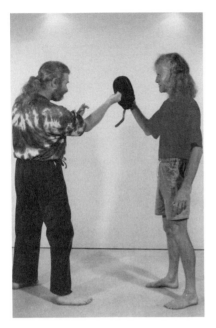

Figure 246

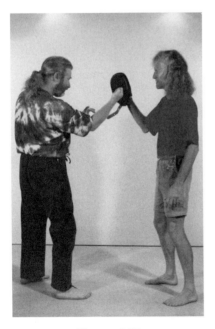

Figure 247

The first training method is for your partner to hold one mitt toward you. You strike the mitt using the same punch that began the first set, only this time you are using the last three knuckles and turning the fist over so it is facing upward upon impact (fig. 246).

This is done with a left/right fa-jing shake of the waist. You do another fa-jing left/right shake, and this time attack with the tiger paw fist facing upward (fig. 247). The two attacks should be done with as little time between each as possible without losing the technique.

THE SAN-SAU
(KUMITE)

This san-sau is directly related to Solo Kata No. 10 in Chapter 10. You have your right foot forward. Your partner attacks with a straight right to your face. You avoid it, as we have done before in the beginning kumite, and attack to his mind point on the left side of the jaw (fig. 248). In the first set we used the tiger paw to Cv 24, but this time we use the last three knuckles and attack the jaw.

Notice that the left palm is snaking over the top of the right wrist. The left palm grabs around the back of his neck as the right tiger paw fist is withdrawn (fig. 249).

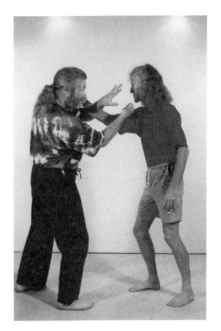

Figure 248

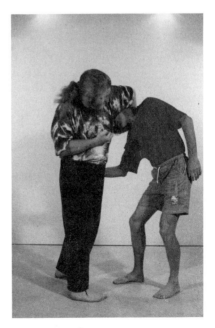

Figure 249

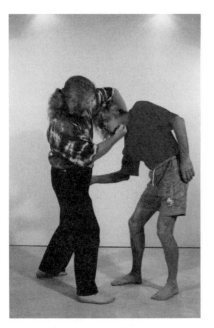

Your left palm pulls him forward onto your right tiger paw into his Cv 22 point, thus causing death (fig. 250).

Your left palm now moves over to your left and slams into the side of his neck at Si 16 point, thus causing massive loss of qi, as your right palm snakes underneath your left palm, ready to again grab around his neck (fig. 251).

Figure 250

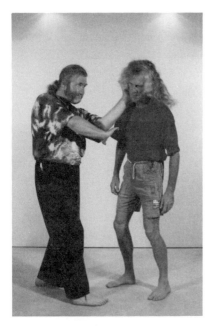

Figure 251

Your right palm pulls his neck down onto your right knee, which is lifted into his neck (fig. 252).

Straight after this, your left palm slams down onto his Small Intestine 1 (Si 1) point located in the center of his scapular, thus weakening his seat of power and so damaging his arm that he would not be able to use it again if he were to survive (fig. 253).

Now take your right foot backward so that the left foot is forward to begin the whole thing on the reverse side.

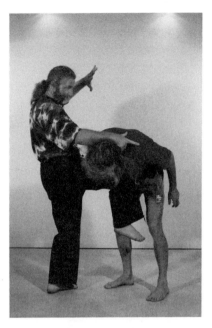

Figure 252

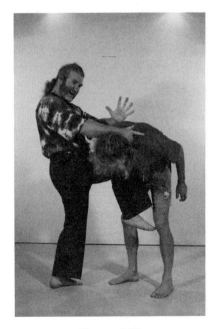

Figure 253

CHAPTER 23

SAN-SAU #11

TRAINING THE HANDS

Your partner holds his right mitt low while his other one is at about face height, pointing downward. Using the power of your waist turning centrifugally (not in a fa-jing way) to your left, you attack the lower mitt with the back of your right palm. Remember that you should use the right side of the back of your palm as the striking area this time (fig. 254).

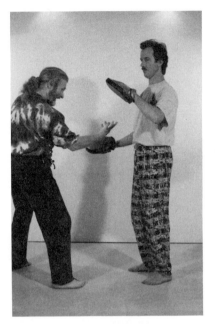

Now you begin the fa-jing. Your waist turns to the right and left violently, taking your right palm upward to strike the second mitt with the backs of your fingers. Be careful with this one at first until you have the technique down. The fingers could be hurt if you do it incorrectly (fig. 255).

Figure 254

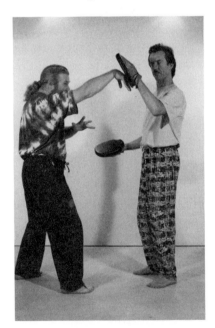

Figure 255

As you turn your waist to your right, your partner turns his right mitt upward so that your right palm can strike down onto it with a clawing motion (fig. 256).

Notice that the left elbow is ready to strike. He turns the mitt so that it is pointing to his right. Using that same turning to the right (waist), you slam the mitt with your left elbow. Both of these strikes use the same turning of the waist, which means that the elbow is only a split second behind the downward palm strike (fig. 257).

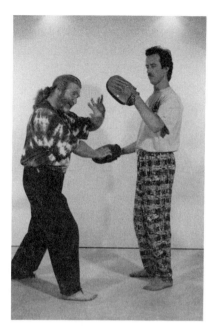

Figure 256

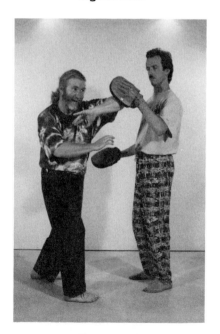

Figure 257

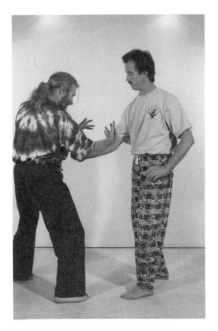

Figure 258

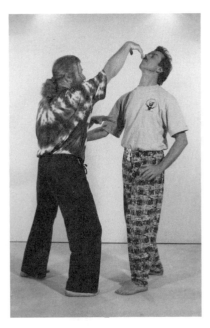

Figure 259

THE SAN-SAU
(KUMITE)

This san-sau is directly related to Solo Kata No. 11 in Chapter 11. Your partner attacks with a mid-level right hook. You have your right foot forward as your right palm slams to the inside of his right elbow just above the elbow (fig. 258). You have used the centrifugal force of your waist turning to your left.

Shake your waist to your right and then to your left as you thrust your right palm (facing downward) up and strike him directly under the nose using the backs of your fingers. The strike is primarily to a point called Gv 26, just under the nose; however, the fingers will probably strike the whole of the front of his face as his head is pushed backward. This strike causes a communication gap between his yin and yang energies, so he becomes scattered and does not know where he is (fig. 259).

Your right "claw" now claws downward into his eye sockets as your waist begins to turn right (fig. 260). The claw is done with a downward thrust into the Stomach 1 (St 1) points at the base of the eye sockets in the middle of the eye. Apart from the obvious eye damage, a strike to these points will also cause him to feel so ill that he will be unable to carry on.

As your waist turns fully to your right, your right palm continues its downward thrust but moves out to your left to control his right arm and to set up your next strike. Your right palm must also scrape the inside of his right upper arm downward away from his body. As this happens, your left elbow strikes the right side of his neck at Si 16, which is a death point (fig. 261).

This whole technique

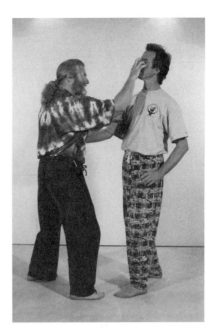

Figure 260

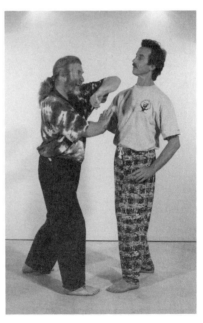

Figure 261

has only taken half a second to execute. It will become easier as you progress. Each of the movements follow one another naturally, hence speed can be generated with this technique in particular.

Now take a left step and do the whole thing on the reverse side.

SAN-SAU #12

TRAINING THE HANDS

With your right foot forward, strike to both mitts using your right hammer fist and your left knife edge. The hammer strikes slightly before the knife edge. Turn your waist to your right as you do this (fig. 262).

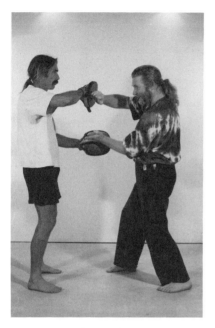

Circle both palms over and strike both mitts again using the hammer and knife edge. Your partner has to turn the mitts so that they face the correct direction (fig. 263).

Figure 262

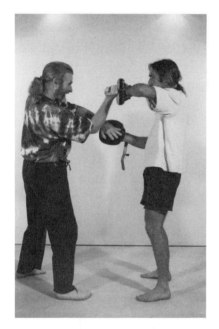

Figure 263

Now your partner turns both mitts toward you as you withdraw both palms and make tiger paw fists with them. You strike both mitts with your fists, the left one leading slightly before the right one (fig. 264).

The last strike (fig. 265) can be done either to a kick bag or to your partner's shoulder. *Don't do it too many times, as his body could be put out of alignment!* Cock your right elbow and turn your waist to your left, then release your elbow and strike with the inside of it (the old clothesline).

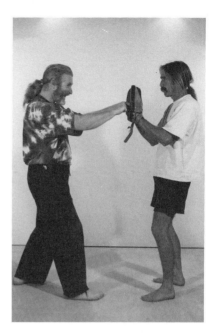

Figure 264

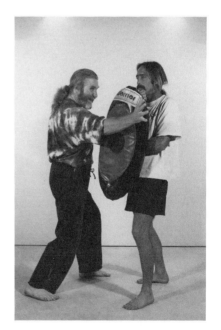

Figure 265

THE SAN-SAU (KUMITE)

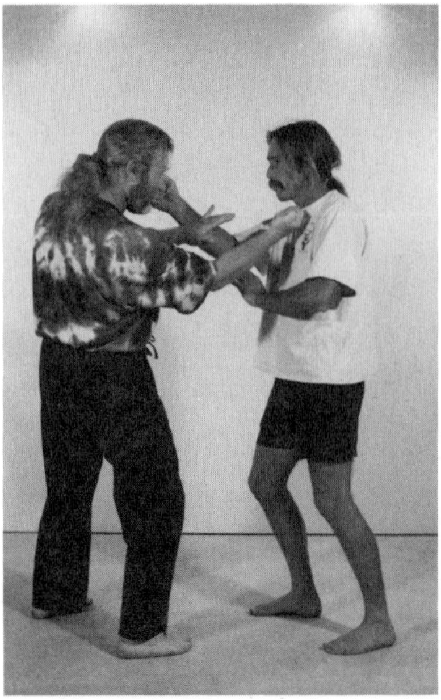

This san-sau is directly related to Solo Kata No. 12 in Chapter 12. Your partner attacks with a straight right to your face. You respond with the same strike that you used in the very first kumite. You avoid his strike by moving your weight to your right and attack to his Gv 26 point just under his nose with your right tiger paw fist (fig. 266).

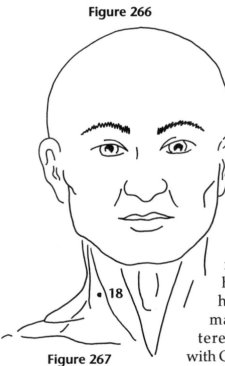

Figure 266

Now rotate both palms so that your right hammer fist will attack his Colon 18 (Co 18) point at the side of his neck, just forward of Small Intestine 16 (fig. 267). As in Figure 268, your left palm (facing up) will attack his Gall Bladder 2 point, just forward of his ear notch (fig. 269). Colon 18 has the effect of detaching his mind from his body, making him totally scattered. Used in conjunction with Gb 2, it will cause death.

Figure 267

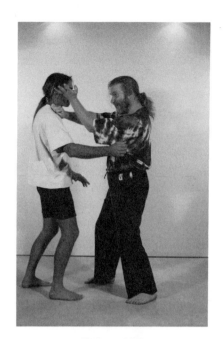

Figure 268

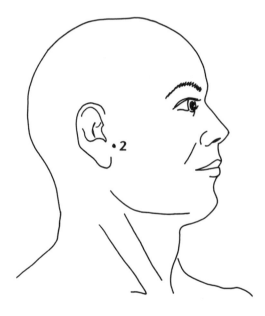

Figure 269

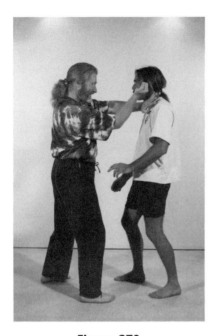

Figure 270

You now reverse your palms so that the left one is facing down and the right fist is palm up. Strike to those same points, Gb 2 and Co 18, as your waist turns to your left (fig. 270).

Pull both palms back slightly and make tiger paw fists. With a quick shake of your waist from left to right, thrust your right tiger paw into the left side of his neck while the left palm is thrust into Cv 22. This combination is a death strike. The right second knuckle is attacking to St 10, which causes the vagus nerve to react violently, thus shutting down the heart (fig. 271).

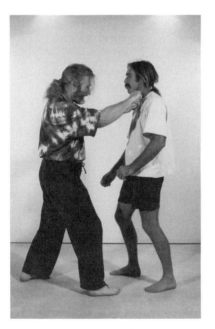

Figure 271

Now grab around the back of his neck with both palms as you drag your right foot back so it's even with your left one. Pull his neck forward violently, thus breaking his neck (fig. 272).

Take a left step forward and out to your left and, with a turning of your waist to your left, slam his neck again with the inside of your right elbow (fig. 273), never giving a sucker an even break! (I said at the beginning that this was the art of overkill!)

You now have your left foot forward to begin the whole set on the reverse side.

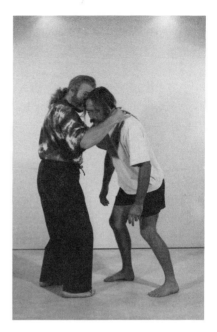

Figure 272

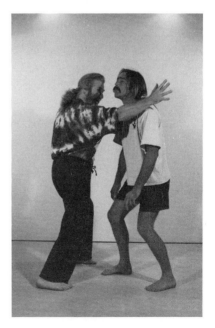

Figure 273

CONCLUSION

Remember, it took 12 years to learn these 12 kata and san-sau. That's how long it takes to master them. The time is well spent, though, as when you have mastered these you will need no other self-defense method. The most deadly techniques ever invented are presented here and must be taken responsibly. I have found, over my many years of teaching, that those who would use these techniques for evil eventually give up, as they just have not the mind for such training. Those who stick it out find that they lean more toward the healing side of dim-mak. And these 12 katas give you the necessary ingredients to be able to become a great healer as well as a great martial artist

As you and your partner become more proficient and begin to "know" each other better, you then begin to make very slight contact—slaps to the face, etc. This is to train each person to be able to take a hit. This is important, as 50 percent of a confrontation is lost or won by being able to take a hit. It is the shock that gets you. Remember, *light contact!* These techniques are dangerous even at a light level of contact.

All of the above is also covered in my video No. MTG621, *The 12 Deadly Katas of Dim-Mak*, available from MTG Video (see page 206).

DIM-MAK'S 12 MOST DEADLY KATAS

ABOUT THE AUTHOR

Erle Montaigue is one of the leading instructors of the internal arts of t'ai chi ch'uan, pa-kua chang, and qigong and is recognized internationally as such. He received the degree of master when he became the first Westerner to perform at the All China National Wushu Tournament in May 1985 and is believed to be the only Westerner to have received such an honor. Erle was tested for hours by three of the world's greatest masters in China. He has been practicing the internal arts since 1968 and is able to trace his lineage in a straight line back to the founder of the Yang style, Yang Lu-Ch'an. He was one of the first students of Chu King-Hung, who was one of the first students of the late Yang Sau-Chung, the eldest son of Yang Cheng-Fu. Erle has had many other great teachers from China as well. He has taught in London, and he is one of the only Westerners to have taught t'ai chi back to the Chinese in Hong Kong in 1981. He now teaches in Australia.

Erle is also one of the main students of Chang Y'iu-Chun, the late student of Yang Shao-Hou. Chang taught Erle the secrets of the original Yang style (old Yang Lu-ch'an style and also the art of dim-mak), which is actually t'ai chi ch'uan.

Erle is the vice chairman of the Federation of Australian Wushu and Kun Gu Organizations and is the course coordinator of the T'ai Chi and Pa-Kua sections of the National Coaching Accreditation Scheme for kung fu. He is also the first t'ai chi person to be given Level Two of the Sports Accreditation Scheme for t'ai chi and pa-kua. This level is considered to be of Olympic standard, if t'ai chi (heaven forbid) were an Olympic sport! He is also president of the Australian Therapeutic Movement Association. This association boasts schools in more than 23 countries, all of which have learned t'ai chi in some way from Erle Montaigue. Erle is also the editor of the magazine *Combat and Healing*, distributed worldwide.

Schools all around the world now use the Erle Montaigue name in their teaching. Erle has taught in Hong Kong, London, and Sydney, Australia, and has given workshops all around the world. Articles authored by Erle Montaigue have appeared in almost every international martial arts magazine, to make t'ai chi and pa-kua the great fighting arts that they are known to be today.

His books are published worldwide, as are his self-teaching videos. People around the world have learned t'ai chi or pa-kua in this way, and they probably never would have been able to do so had it not been for these videos. Many of the world's leading karate teachers, as high as sixth dan, have learned from Erle's videos and attended his workshops.

Before t'ai chi kung fu, Erle Montaigue was well versed in the Western art of amateur and professional wrestling, which he now brings into his classes as an adjunct to the kung fu training. Erle is also an accomplished modern musician, having had albums recorded under his name.

He now travels to the United States, Canada, and Europe twice per year to teach martial arts, as well as leading workshops in New Zealand and Australia

Erle Montaigue has a large selection of videos covering every possible aspect of the martial/healing arts, including taiji, dim-mak, bagwa, qigong, iron shirt qigong, weapons, and the Montaigue system. If you would like a free catalog of these titles, please write to:

MTG VIDEO
P.O. Box 792
Murwillumbah NSW 2484
Australia
Fax: (your overseas code) + 61-66-797028